Once Upon a *Wishbone*

Michele Wachter

Once Upon a *Wishbone*

*Finding Light Through a Story of Hope,
Connection and Rediscovered Purpose*

PALMETTO
PUBLISHING
Charleston, SC
www.PalmettoPublishing.com

Copyright © 2024 by Michele Wachter

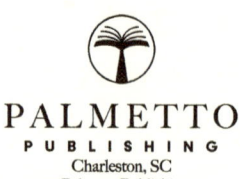

All rights reserved
No portion of this book may be reproduced, stored in a retrieval system, or transmitted in any form by any means–electronic, mechanical, photocopy, recording, or other–except for brief quotations in printed reviews, without prior permission of the author.

Hardcover ISBN: 9798822978522
Paperback ISBN: 9798822978539

The content contained within this book may not be reproduced, duplicated or transmitted without direct written permission from the author or the publisher.

Under no circumstances will any blame or legal responsibility be held against the publisher, or author, for any damages, reparation, or monetary loss due to the information contained within this book, either directly or indirectly.

Legal Notice:

This book is copyright protected. It is only for personal use. You cannot amend, distribute, sell, use, quote or paraphrase any part, or the content within this book, without the consent of the author or publisher.

Disclaimer Notice:

Please note the information contained within this document is for educational and entertainment purposes only. All effort has been executed to present accurate, up to date, reliable, complete information. No warranties of any kind are declared or implied. Readers acknowledge that the author is not engaged in the rendering of legal, financial, medical or professional advice. The content within this book has been derived from various sources. Please consult a licensed professional before attempting any techniques outlined in this book.

By reading this document, the reader agrees that under no circumstances is the author responsible for any losses, direct or indirect, that are incurred as a result of the use of the information contained within this document, including, but not limited to, errors, omissions, or inaccuracies.

Table of Contents

About the Author..i
Preface iii
Content Warning.. vii
Introduction..ix

Chapter 1: The Rejection 1
    The Dream... 1
    An Ode to My Grandma 2
    Separated Forever.................................... 3
    The Dream Grows: Catholic School..................... 4
    The Dream Shatters: My First Rejection............... 5
    Lost 5
    The Safe Path: Marriage.............................. 6
    In a Nutshell: The Turbulence of the Early Years 6
    In Hindsight 7

Chapter 2: Finally, a Calling 9
    Marriage: A Blessing................................ 10
    The Story of My Father............................. 11
    Loveless Reunions 12
    My Marriage Goes South 13
    Two Years Later... Finally, Answers 15
    The No-Brainer Decision............................ 17
    Work Begins.. 18
    Another Setback... Or Blessing?.................... 20

An Ode to My Mother..........................20
　　In a Nutshell: Finding My Feet..................21
　　In Hindsight.................................22

Chapter 3: My Time with Mr. E....................23
　　Meeting the Man Who Changed My Life..........23
　　Breakthroughs...............................25
　　Down Memory Lane...........................27
　　Gaining Momentum...........................33
　　Further Headway.............................37
　　In a Nutshell: My Time with Mr. E...............39
　　In Hindsight.................................40

Chapter 4: New Beginnings.........................41
　　A Failing Marriage............................41
　　Final Straws.................................43
　　A Life of Separation..........................44
　　The Work Front..............................45
　　In a Nutshell: The Year 2009...................47
　　In Hindsight.................................48

Chapter 5: Farewell, Mr. E.........................49
　　Declining Health.............................50
　　The End Draws Near..........................51
　　Shiva.......................................52
　　In His Memory...............................53
　　In a Nutshell: The Passing.....................53
　　In Hindsight.................................54

Chapter 6: The Owl and the Promise 55
   Wherein I Try (and Fail) to Move On. 55
   A Memory of Love That No One Can Steal 57
   The Promise. 58
   In a Nutshell: My Calling, Renewed. 58
   In Hindsight 59

Chapter 7: The Start of Something Beautiful. 61
   Hopes and Prayers 62
   The Seeds of Love 63
   Wedding Bells 64
   In a Nutshell: Marriage and Settlement 65
   In Hindsight 65

Chapter 8: Looking Ahead 67
   Life Continues: Gaining Further Expertise. 68
   Volunteer Work Continues. 68
   Plans for the Future: Aiming for the Stars. 69
   Passing the Torch 70
   In a Nutshell: Settling Down 72
   In Hindsight 73

Chapter 9: The Joys of a Life Well Lived 75
   Realizations 76
   The Cup Is Always Half Full 77
   Family: A Blessing Not to be Underestimated. 78
   Mr. E: My Best Friend 83
   For Bosses and Workplaces. 83
   For Forgiveness and Reconciliation. 84
   The Dream That Came True 85
   In a Nutshell: Joys and Gratitude 85
   In Hindsight 86

Chapter 10: Tools & Techniques to Treat Dementia 87
    The Origins of Care 88
    With Understanding Comes Compassion 89
    Enter Their Stories with Them 90
    Laughter as a Medicine 91
    Recreation is Key: Get 'em Outta the House 91
    A Sense of Purpose 92
    Role Reversals 92
    Old Memories 93
    The Power of Conviction 94
    Non-Verbal Cues 94
    Non-Verbal Instructions 95
    In a Nutshell: Caring in the Time of Dementia 96
    In Hindsight 96

Chapter 11: Client Success Stories 97
    #1 The Power of Old Memories 98
    #2 Discovering Mystery Triggers 100
    #3 Role Reversals 102
    #4 Non-Verbal Instructions 103
    #5 Using the Power of Conviction 104
    #6 A Combination: Recreation, Purpose, and Role Reversals . . 105
    Steps to Take 106
    In a Nutshell: Cases That Stood Out 108
    In Hindsight 108

Conclusion 111
References 113

About the Author

Michele Wachter is experienced in caring for clients with Alzheimer's and other dementias. She is based in Long Island, New York and has been working with the elderly since she was a small child. With her congenital missing left hand, she has learned to battle life single-handedly. With experience as a full-time mom, she is also experienced in the art of managing tantrums, accidents, events, and much more. Juggling voluntary service, her job as a caregiver/trainer, and her personal practice, she's also an expert at multitasking. With these well-rounded, super-charged skills in her repertoire, Michele adds her singular passion for caring and giving back to the community as a final ingredient to her care routines. Michele has worked as a hands-on caregiver for years, improving her techniques individually as she went on.

Since 2011, Michele has also excelled as a trainer for other caregivers and aides, imparting her knowledge to enable them in their respective fields. As life finally gives her some room to breathe, she has turned her attention to recording the events of her life that led her to this point and to inspiring others through her highly unconventional journey. In doing this, she lays out her heart and the circumstances of her life for others to see and learn from, much as she lays out the secrets and tricks of the trade that she's acquired over years of practice, research, and teaching. These tips are currently alive in her trainees as they spread her knowledge and love.

Today, Michele is working as an advisor for professional caregivers and family members who want her signature out-of-the-box solutions and advice to create personalized care plans for Alzheimer's clients. Her startup is called "Empowering Professionals in Dementia Care, LLC." It bears the emblem of an owl, a symbol she holds close to her heart as a promise to a loved one: a promise that she will give her very best to her clients, always.

Michele's journey continues as she flourishes, but she writes this book now to record a moment that she wishes to encapsulate in her memory forever and everything that led to it.

Preface

In the halls of memory, echoes laugh
A symphony of old joys and photographs
In every corner, a story told
Of old days of silver and nights of gold
Yesteryears' shadows, long and lean,
Dance in the dusk, unseen, serene.
So let us wander through the corridors of time,
Where laughter echoes and bells softly chime
For in memories' embrace, we find solace and grace
A bittersweet dance of past and present's embrace —Phrysylla

With a profession in dealing with and protecting others' memories, this book was a necessary step for me: It's where I recollect my Suitcase of Memories, as I call it, collecting things that are important to me. After all, it's by force of habit that I store stories. This one happens to be my own, with snippets of the lives that touched mine deeply. It's where I put down what I learned and how I learned it, what I gave to others and the gratification and experience that I gained in return.

As I approach stability in my career as a geriatric caregiver for Alzheimer's clients and a certified trainer for other professional aides, caregivers, and companions, I often look back at the unique circumstances that led me to these heights. With over 20 years of experience, I wanted to lay out the essence of my years of service. This book is a self-reflective collection of anecdotes and circumstances that taught and nurtured me, cultivating and polishing me into the person I am today. It's also an example for others who may be struggling to find their feet. Reader, if this is you, then I can deeply sympathize, but I know that you'll get through!

As I thought about my life, I realized that my path had been highly unconventional, getting my experience well before I got my certification. Moreover, it was riddled with additional problems from being born without a left hand, a circumstance outside my control that pushed me off the normal route. All of this taught me a great deal, and I felt that my story could help others who feel lost because they're off the mainstream track. A lot of this book is about the different ways I was lost throughout my life. However, I believe that we're all on different paths that lead to our destined purpose, so whatever profession you're aiming for, if you're floundering, it means that you're learning and being prepared and toughened up for much better. In presenting my story, I hope that it finds people who need to hear real stories of someone else who kept losing their way until they found the right one.

Among the elements that honed me and encouraged my abilities, my family and friends are foremost. Any recollections about the past make my heart swell with love and pride and gratitude, and I knew that, before anything else, I needed to publish an ode to the gems I met and the gems I'm honored to have been raised with because, without them, I would be incomplete. A major purpose of this book, therefore, is to act as a token of love for my companions in life.

From a lost young lady missing a left hand to a successful trainer starting my own business, life threw many curveballs and hurdles to prepare me for my position. And now that I'm preparing to pass the torch and impart what I learned, I wanted to share my journey and its challenges. In these stories tucked safely in the attic of my mind, I believe one can find the reasons behind my passion for caregiving. This is essential because once you find your *why*, the *how* becomes simpler. So, one facet of this book is self-reflection and self-discovery, putting down what I know about myself to find things I may have missed. As I unpack my life, you, too, can choose things to learn from and mistakes to avoid.

Finally, as Dutch Resistance fighter Corrie Ten Boom put it, "Memories are the key not to the past, but to the future" (Watson, 2015). Now, as I launch my own business in consultative services for professional aides and loving caregivers for people with dementia, I seek to put down my memories as keys to future caregivers. In them are hints to the kinds of love and support one can seek to drive them through caregiving and practical ways in which I balanced my practical and personal life. It also has a recollection of how I learned to give quality care to my clients and how I improved, hoping to inspire readers who are still in the difficult, initial phases.

In short, I believe that the best way to teach is through examples and demonstrations, and my life is one story that I can recount to do both things. All at once, it's an ode to those who touched me, a self-reflection on things that taught and honed me, and a guide for those who want to enter the field or can benefit from my experiences. It's my Suitcase of Memories.

Content Warning

This book refers to religions, specifically Catholic Christianity and Judaism, as a part of the main characters' lives. It does not, however, attempt to preach either religion; the tone remains narrative. Any prejudices or discrimination has been avoided, and all opinions are personal.

The book also refers to congenital defects and parental abandonment, but there are no graphic details of either; it is merely a part of my narrative.

Introduction

Once Upon a Wishbone tracks my life from my birth to where I currently stand, ending with an introduction to the business I am currently launching. As the title suggests, the story is almost like a miracle–a fairy tale where my childhood dream came true years after I lost my path. A comprehensive index of my life, this book records and presents key moments and feelings that led to the decisions I made and which shaped my story.

The first seven chapters of this book follow my life in fairly chronological order, stopping briefly to give odes to key people in my life. In these chapters, you can follow my initial stages as a child born without her left hand and abandoned by her father, only to find her calling at the impressionable age of six. It then follows me through the rejection of this dream, a failing marriage, and three daughters as I tried and (as I thought when I couldn't see immediate results) failed to achieve the kind of success I wanted from life. With this recollection, I follow my path through finally finding my place in the profession I'd always wanted, becoming a certified Alzheimer's caregiver and trainer to other caregivers, family members, and professionals in the geriatric industry. I then recount the joy of getting married to the man of my dreams and of meeting wonderful people along the way. This section gives a realistic narration of my life, reading like a story from my point of view.

The following two chapters are opposites. One is in retrospect, giving an overview and an ode to the amazing people I met and lived with and the things I'm grateful for, from the bitter lessons to the sweet memories. The other is an optimistic account of where I stand in life today and where I hope to be in the future. These two chapters are mostly self-reflective and give an insight into how much these people mean to me.

Finally, I have included snippets and six case studies of former clients with general tools and techniques for dealing with Alzheimer's clients. This section aims to act as a guide for readers who know or who are caring for such clients and need out-of-the-box solutions. It also gives tips on how to look for such solutions. Since every client needs a personalized care routine, the "how to do it" becomes more important than the "what to do" unless I know your client. Therefore, these chapters are a sneak-peek training round and an insider-tip session.

As every chapter ends, you'll find an "In a Nutshell" section that summarizes key points in the chapter, followed by an "In Hindsight" section. The former closes each chapter of my life's path, to be read as a conclusive reflection on different points in my memoir. The latter is devoted to how this chapter in my life impacted my career as a geriatric care provider/trainer. This section is for existing or aspiring caregivers, demonstrating what I learned throughout my career and how I learned it.

Right at the end of *Once Upon a Wishbone*, you'll find a little section about my business as a trainer for other caregivers. If you want first-hand advice or tips, here's where you can get them! Watch out for details in the final pages.

Readers, I'm honored that you've picked up this book, and I'm extremely excited to share the story of my life. So, without further ado, let's begin!

Chapter 1:
The Rejection

When I was a little girl, fairy tales were my favorite books because even before you opened them you knew how they were going to end - happily ever after. –Nicola Yoon

My story begins, perhaps, when I was born. After all, this was when the nurse first saw that my left hand was missing and that I wouldn't ever be a "normal," complete child. But even then, my soul was whole. I was normal for all I knew and cared about. Thus, I came into the world a healthy child, but with a single condition that, little did I know back then, would break and remake my dream.

Therefore, perhaps my story begins when I was first aware of this fateful dream. When I, too, made a wish like the innocent child that opens a fairy tale and believes, no, *expects* their fairy godmother and magic to save the day and make dreams come true. And this happened on a day that remains carved into my memory.

The Dream

It was an extraordinary day in my mostly ordinary life: the auspicious date that marked the sixth year since I was born without my left hand. And as for any loved child who lived in her grandmother's warm, comfortable arms, there was a party. In our little celebration, there was a wishbone that I can recall: a little, delicate thing that a little, six-year-old princess could wish upon and break with her delicate, precious hands.

Only, in my case, of course, there was only one hand. But this was a fact I wasn't made aware of so strongly, because I always had my beloved Grandma holding the other end of the wishbone.

We gripped opposite ends of the bone. My blue eyes locked with those beloved chestnut brown ones as my petite, slender hand felt the warmth of those soft, leathery, gentle ones covered in the sweet scent of lotion and wrinkled with age. Stray locks of her dark brown hair framed her face, and I felt at home.

In this setting of pure comfort and love, we made our wishes.

As I thought of what to wish for, my grandmother wished that I'd grow up to be a nurse just as I was her "Little Nurse." As I felt the warmth of her love, I wished for the same: to be a nurse when I grew up, so I could care for other lovable treasure troves of experience like Grandma.

Mark Twain once said, "The two most important days in life are the day you are born and the day you find out why" (Seybold, 2016, para. 2). For me, the two were six years apart. Because on that fateful day, sitting in the warmth of my grandma's little kitchen, I made a potent wish that would stay with me throughout my life. Even now, it marks the beginning of The Dream That Came True.

An Ode to My Grandma

As I grew up, I was extremely lucky to be surrounded by people I loved and who loved me. We lived in a cozy, loving, two-family house, with myself, my parents, and my brother Michael, who I called "Moon," living upstairs.

Downstairs, with my grandfather, lived a person I loved with my heart and soul: my grandmother. She became one of the most influential people in my life after my father abandoned us when I was five–a year before I made my wish. As I learned to help her with her agoraphobia and heart problems, I learned to care for the elderly. Grandma left her loving embrace deeply embedded in my memories as I continued to love other senior people, including her friends Lilly and Eloise. Perhaps they reminded me of her. Or perhaps she, at 60, had helped me find my calling at the young and impressionable age of six.

Separated Forever

To this date, I remember the warmth of Grandma's lips as she kissed me goodbye and whispered, "I love you, Shell."

That was the last I saw of her before the ambulance drove away. The next day, May 18th, 1980, she left us forever. In my devastation, I remember 7-year-old me sobbing at her casket, "Grandma, who is going to make me my oatmeal with rainbow sprinkles and a cup of Sanka coffee?"

I knew we'd never again get to have our daily breakfast together. Even as I write this, my heart still sinks at the thought of this devastating loss.

After all, Grandma and I were best friends. She was my source of comfort, and I was the light of her eyes. Little did I know that she'd inspire me to return to caring for seniors and become a professional in the field!

After Grandma left, I stayed close to her friends and my childhood best friend, Danielle. Through Danielle's grandmother Gertie, I also had my first exposure to Alzheimer's back in 1982, when I was just ten years old. Gertie was diagnosed with the disease when she was 50, and I still remember her as a loving, kind woman: a grandmother that any child could wish for. As time passed, I remained friends with Danielle, her motivating words driving me on whenever my promise to Grandma threatened to weaken.

On the other hand, I also had Grandma's other friends as people to love and care for. This, too, would go on to fuel my passion for working with the elderly, especially ones with Alzheimer's.

The Dream Grows: Catholic School

For 13 blissful years of my life, I'd gone to a private Catholic school. Grandma was Italian by birth, and our family was centered around familial love and religion. My mother wanted me to learn about God and to be in a smaller setting where I wouldn't be bullied over my missing left hand. I was lucky. I was given the freedom to wish and dream. And so, the wish–or promise, perhaps–that I'd made with Grandma a year before she passed away continued to burn like an ember in my heart.

During these years, my mother was my biggest cheerleader. She raised me to never give up as she worked tirelessly to provide for my brother and me. I'd seen her wearing herself thin, and I wanted to emulate her. She's the strongest woman I know. As her daughter, I had what it took to live my dream. I could do what it took to become a nurse!

I knew what I'd love to do, and I knew that I wouldn't be able to let it go without giving it a shot in the professional world.

The Dream Shatters: My First Rejection

In 1992, I was finally almost ready to enter the nursing program. I entered the public City College, ecstatic that I was close to attaining my dream. All was well.

"Was" is the keyword, because then I sat with the nursing advisor to cover the formalities. I wanted to be transparent with her, telling her clearly about my congenital defect. I assured her that I could do everything the others could. I told her that I had my mother's support and my childhood dream behind me. But all while I spoke, I watched her face fall, and I could feel the doom approach. I watched as it neared the surface like you watch a boiling saucepan of curry, its froth rising and rising until it splashes upon the stove that had been squeaky clean a moment earlier. And erupt it did, upon the squeaky-clean surface of my long-held hopes when the advisor finally spoke: I'd need both my hands to handle the rigor of being a nurse.

The conversation had a dreadful air of finality to it. I wouldn't be able to follow my dream and passion professionally.

Lost

After years of harboring the dream I'd had since I was six, I was shattered. It was as if I'd only asked for one thing in life: to help the elderly. Now I'd have to change my goals in life and find myself again. I was floundering in self-doubt and hopelessness.

For two years, I tried to find the light again. I had to pick up the broken pieces and see what I could do to find my new purpose in life. And then I decided I'd marry my childhood sweetheart, who was successful in his field as a police officer. It helped that he wanted me to stay at home and care for the family. The relationship wasn't the healthiest, but I wasn't particularly ready to replace my passion for nursing with anything else, anyway. I was fine as a housewife. Plus, he'd been my sweetheart since I'd been sixteen, so what could go wrong?

Life was guiding me toward a new path. I took it.

The Safe Path: Marriage

For quite a few years, I found solace in marriage and having kids. They were dependent on me, and I loved loving and caring for them. I loved cooking and cleaning and fulfilling my role as a mother and wife. I found joy in my kids' little faces as they called me "Mom." Like a balm, it filled the gaping hole left by my nursing dream.

For a few blissful years, I found some semblance of peace.

In a Nutshell: The Turbulence of the Early Years

My early life was riddled with misfortunes, most importantly, abandonment from my father, the lack of a left hand, and the loss of Grandma. However, I still consider those years some of the best in my life.

I believe that, for a child, two things are the most important: to feel safe and to be loved. Thanks to Grandma's memory and her friends, I was loved. Thanks to my mother's deep love and ever-ready support and the Catholic school's nonjudgmental, welcoming culture, I felt safe. Add to that Grandma's friends and a loyal, supportive confidante like Danielle, and I had company, both in my age group and above it. I had a playmate and wells of wisdom, both within reach. To top it all off, I had a dream–a purpose in life that I kept as a talisman in my heart, keeping me going through it all.

It was as I grew up that I was exposed to the darker side of the world and experienced disappointment. You see, as long as a child feels safe and loved, they can comprehend and accept loss. But when they feel betrayed or misunderstood or when they feel as if they're being kept away from their full potential, that's when they truly feel lost. And when I lost my vision, I suppose that's when I felt utterly handicapped and dejected for the first time.

In Hindsight

Fast forwarding to the future years, this is a principle I work on a great deal: for the elderly, too, stability and love matter. As long as they receive these, they can handle the rest.

When I joined the field, I tried to give my clients what Grandma once gave me–and I still do.

Chapter 2:
Finally, a Calling

It's not enough to have lived. We should be determined to live for something. —Leo Buscaglia

After I got married, my struggle to find who I was supposed to be continued. I knew for sure that I loved caring for people. It gratified me to see their joy. But my mind had questions even when my heart (on the surface, at least!) told me that my life full:

What kind of love and care would fill me up so potently that I could do it all my life?

What did I want to see in return?

Was I willing to care for someone who did not reciprocate?

You see, you can never really silence the inner voice that questions you. The problem is when its questions are valid, the answers are within reach, and you choose to ignore them for the greater good. As long as that greater good remains, you hold the questions at bay, but the minute it stops acting as a barrier, the flood you've been damming in gushes out in full force. I was afraid of a flood that would destroy everything; I needed an outlet to slowly let the water out and, with it, the pressure.

This chapter of my life was wrought with questions. After all, from the age of six I'd known exactly what I wanted from life, and now I'd lost it. It would take me a long time to fully accept my new role.

Marriage: A Blessing

A marriage made with love is supposed to be a beautiful union where each finds solace and support in the other. And so was mine - at first.

What could be better than marrying your high school sweetheart who's been there for you since you were sixteen? Steven held my hand when I was at the lowest point in my life, supported me, and pulled me out of my listlessness. He was perfect. Plus, he was three years older than me so he was mostly settled. Floundering as I was, I leaped at the chance to be settled with him.

This was why I married him. And I loved my Steven. He made up for my flaws and drawbacks because he had a job, whereas I'd failed at my dream career. He wanted me to stay at home when I didn't have the courage to find another career. And he gave me my lovely kids who became the light, purpose, and joy of my life. It was a beautiful union! I didn't regret not having my career. I didn't look back—not once. Or so I said to myself, anyway.

And then, at 23, I had my first child: my daughter, Jillian. The moment I looked into her adorable eyes, held her delicate, soft, tiny hands, and felt that baby skin, I felt as if my heart would burst with joy. I was full of love and the powerful instinct to protect and nurture the precious gift I had been given. The feeling was potent. The emotions were fulfilling. I was content. I was happy.

As Jillian grew up, my life was full of all that a mother cherishes about her child. I was cooking, cleaning, teaching, and learning how to be a mother. I was in the Nursing School of Life, and I was practicing as I went along. My little Jill was my flesh and blood; she was the apple of my eye. Her childish innocence and the way she smiled up at me won my heart so thoroughly that I felt I'd give everything up for this little creature. I hadn't felt love this unconditional, this pure and strong and dependable, since Grandma had passed. Now, I had a similar bond with Jill. She even had the same chestnut brown hair as Grandma! The fact that Jill overall looked like Steven with her hair and her little brown eyes only added to my determination to keep her with her father as long as I could.

Living to absorb my daughter's first words, her darling smile, her baby steps, and her fast-growing little fingerprints smearing chocolate and cookie dough across my squeaky-clean walls (I loved cleaning!), I lived Cinderella's life, minus the wicked stepmother, plus Prince Charming, singing contentedly in my own little palace, away from the World Beyond. And if I sometimes sang of the dream that is a wish the heart makes when you're fast asleep, I didn't think much of it.

Any questions I had about the wisdom of abandoning my dream over a nursing advisor's opinion were silenced for a while longer. Until, of course, my textbook fairytale hit a taste of reality.

The Story of My Father

Remember when I mentioned my father? Well, I didn't like mentioning him much back then, either. But as I felt my heart swell with pride and joy at my darling daughter, I wondered what he had felt when he'd seen me. Did he love me? Did he have the same urge to pick me up and twirl me around until we both collapsed in a laughing mess on the ground? Did he ever hug me tight and want to protect me from the world outside? Was I so precious to him?

How did he manage to walk away when I was just five? Because I clearly remember the day he left me: a year before I wished I could care for the elderly all my life. It was my fifth birthday when he'd abandoned us. I was slightly older than Jill was now (she'd just turned four). I woke up and, instead of a party, I found out that my father had left.

As a little girl who still hoped for a little magic, I waited for him. I waited as days turned into nights, and my father, the alcoholic that he was, never came back. Growing up, I'd often listen to the song "Somewhere Out There" and look up into the sky, deep into the stars that were the same for me and my father. I'd pray that he'd be thinking about me, too. And then my heart would break again when he didn't come back.

I cried. And I withdrew and turned to Grandma for comfort, because she truly loved me.

Perhaps, now that I think about it, my passion for caring for others stemmed from my relationship with Dad. Psychologically, they say, your childhood affects who you become as an adult. Perhaps I was so desperate to give others love and support because I never had Dad's love as I grew up. And perhaps I chose to do it for the elderly because that's where I found my support system when I had no other.

Nevertheless, enough rambling in retrospect! I was there for Jillian, and I'd protect her from the world as much as I could like my mother had done for me. Until, of course, Life dealt me a curveball that truly left me stumped. My father returned.

Loveless Reunions

As I said, Jillian was 4, and I was 27, when, in the year 2000, I met my father again. He was 61 years old, 5 feet 11 inches tall. He wasn't the strong, powerful man from my dreams, though. He was gaunt, weighing only 80 pounds and shrunken with years of alcoholism and homelessness.

My father didn't recognize me when I walked into the hospital where he lay sick. He never got to play with my Jill. My heart broke once again. I relived the pain of my father's abandonment and was five years old again, wondering why my father had chosen the bottle over us. It was almost more than I could bear. In fact, perhaps it *would* be too much if I didn't have a daughter of my own to protect.

After three weeks of not knowing what to say to or how to feel about my biological father, he passed away. At his wake, I started to pray to the Lord to help me find my purpose once more because my father had brought with him a dark reminder of how a man could abandon his family. I wanted to be independent enough to support my darling. I didn't want my kids to watch their father walk away; I wanted a settlement. I wanted to be strong like my mother.

In the end, I forgave my father because I loved him. As they say, blood is indeed thicker than water. However, I needed to be ready to face the realities I had grown up with because you *can* love someone and be aware of their flaws. Such was the case with my memories of my father.

My Marriage Goes South

Although my marriage with my sweetheart began with bliss and love, it started to disintegrate after a while. He was getting possessive and controlling, and I was unhappy living with him.

Here's a sneak peek: In 2007 (two years after this chapter ends), I returned to college. We were doing a spiritual course about self. The professor put on a scene from *The Lion King*, where Simba loses his identity after losing his father and is unable to take the throne as Mufasa's rightful successor. At this point, his father appears as an apparition to guide him back. I remember bursting into uncontrollable tears, sobbing hysterically because I, too, had lost my identity in my marriage. But in my case, the spirit of Grandma wouldn't return from the dead to say, "Remember who you are."

I, too, felt lost in the desert, alone in my own kingdom, where I had to re-learn the meaning of "Hakuna Matata" and not worry.

With Steven, I did not have any time to myself, nor did my feelings matter to him. All I had were expectations: to manage the house as if my life depended on it and to be there for the kids. *I* was nobody.

Now, having seen my father, I was even more desperate for a way out of the union before our differences had gone too far for us to even reach a peaceful separation for our kids' sake.

However, as much as I wanted to end the marriage safely, I had no career. There was no money, and I wasn't confident enough to take on the role of a single mother and financial provider. I was floundering once more, desperately missing the career I'd wished to have. How ever would I manage?

Only fate would tell.

While I figured out the state of my marriage with Steven, it seems the Lord gave me an answer in the form of my second daughter, Kimberlyanna. She was born on June 8th, 2001. I stuck with my marriage to give them a stable home for as long as I could and tried to find contentment in my domestic life once more. I continued letting my daughters' joy and love and trust become mine, too, and I found some peace in my busy life as a full-time mom.

Kim would grow up to be a natural caregiver, following in my footsteps just as she shared my appearance. Hard as it was staying in the marriage, my children were every bit worth the patience.

Two Years Later… Finally, Answers

With Kim and Jill as my responsibilities and still looking beyond the limits of my marriage, I started asking the Lord for answers again. Once again, I felt that I couldn't make the marriage work. I'd tried for years, through two children and multiple arguments, all ending in me feeling defeated and dejected all over again. I was getting desperate.

Plus, meeting my father had reminded me why a woman should be strong and independent and how my mother had struggled to raise us alone. I also realized that I felt lost in my marriage. I was tied to a man like my mother had been, and I knew how they could leave you high and dry. On top of that, when I was at the hospital with my father, I had a fresh taste of the life I'd always wanted to have as a nurse. With all this in mind, I prayed and watched for answers.

And then, one fine afternoon, as I sat with a local newspaper in my hand and a refreshing mug of coffee on the table, I read something. And then I sat up a little straighter, held the paper a little closer to my face and read it again, more slowly this time. After years of chasing contentment and peace, something new started to spread tiny, cautious roots in my fast-emptying heart, filling it up with something different. Something I hadn't had for years. Something strong rather than tender, fierce like the love I had for my daughters. I felt hope. The hope you get when you see a distant piece of land after months at sea. The hope when you have even a meager tether to guide you home. This, reader, was the power of having the hope of purpose once more.

The advertisement that I'd read in the paper was from Home Instead, an organization for at-home care for elderly people. It was big and bold and seemed tailored to me.

"Do you like seniors?" it asked.

Hell, yeah!

"We're looking for individuals that will be a friend and companion to the seniors," it went on.

Totally up my street! That's literally what I'd been doing in my childhood!

"Job duties: Meal prep, laundry, transportation to doctor's appointments, recreational activities, and listening to their stories," it read.

Tell that to a mother of two! [eyeroll] *Managing one old person was going to be a walk in the park. Literally and figuratively.*

For a few moments, I sat and looked at the paper, hope dangerously and cautiously creeping through my bloodstream, my heart beating a tiny bit faster as I considered the offer carefully. It seemed to be the answer to my dreams. Financial stability and independence in the field that I was passionate about. To top it off, I didn't need to be a certified nurse or have any other professional prerequisites. It seemed too good to be true.

However, as the euphoria wore off, more practical considerations invaded my mind. What would I tell my hubby? He'd particularly wanted a stay-at-home wife. As it was, it seemed I was walking on eggshells around him all the time. How would he react? Plus, I'd have to leave my kids behind every day as I cared for this person. Did that make me a bad mother? Of course, I'd still be doing the housework when I got home and doing my best as their mom. But I might still miss their schooldays and wouldn't be there all the time for them. I was torn.

The No-Brainer Decision

Reader, I chose hope. I chose financial independence and stability. I chose my kids' futures over any present inconveniences and my husband's wishes.

I took the job.

As soon as I made this decision, other things started falling into place, as well. My mind was racing at a million miles per minute, almost like a bird freed from the bars of its cage for the first time. I'd reconnect with Grandma's friends and ask if they wanted to hire me as help. I'd pour life and soul into the elderly people this organization asked me to care for, and I'd rise through the ranks. I'd earn my kids the life I wanted for them. I'd be free from this marriage and become a force to be reckoned with. I had already seen Gertie with her Alzheimer's anyway; I already had experience. It couldn't be too hard, could it? My dream would come true.

As I visualized the future, I felt happy and free. I hugged my daughters in relief, knowing that change was on its way.

Thus, in February 2003, my geriatric career began.

Work Begins

My First Client: Mrs. Helen

Beginning work as a companion for the elderly, I was assigned to my 85-year-old client, my first Alzheimer's disease client. A tiny, frail lady with extremely thick glasses, Mrs. Helen was eccentric, to say the least. For one, she'd always lay the table for three even though she lived alone. She spoke of all the people she knew, but it seemed she didn't know anybody in the present. Whatever was she thinking?

Then, as I got to know my client, and Alzheimer's, better, I started to piece things together. It was like a mystery story where I had to figure out how all the pieces fit. The three place settings, I found, included one for her husband who had passed away from Alzheimer's five years prior. The other was for her daughter. Every day, she prepared in the hope that they'd return for dinner, but they never did. In her mind, her daughter was still the little six-year-old they'd adopted, still living with them, and her husband was alive. She'd almost role-play the day they'd adopted the girl, saying, "I love your red phone" as if she were the child.

With Alzheimer's, you see, a person can live in the past at a particular moment they remember. For Mrs. Helen, one such moment was a delightful dinner she'd had with her parents, talking about them as if they were still alive years after they'd passed away. On another shift, we visited "The Red Door," as she called it. This turned out to be the old Friendly's ice cream parlor where she once ate with her daughter and granddaughter. With incidents like these, I'd have to piece the puzzle together as I learned to jump into their world and join them where they were in their stories.

Perhaps, at some point, it was a welcome relief from my own present to be a part of the best of someone else's past.

On the other hand, there were also bittersweet memories. At Mrs. Helen's place, every day was Christmas. She loved her fiber optic Christmas tree that played music that we'd dance to together, watching its lights change colors. Sad as it was that her family wasn't there to give her the company she so desperately needed, it was gratifying to watch her joy as I accompanied her.

I began to see the beauty in my job, right from the outset.

My Second Client: Ms. Eileen

With Ms. Eileen, another client diagnosed with Alzheimer's, we would take rides and walk together. She loved talking about her kids and grandkids. However, once, when her best friend for many years visited us, Ms. Eileen accused that friend of stealing her underwear. A conversation like this ensued:

An offended, "I'd never steal her underwear; I'm twice her size!"

And then, proceeding to hold Ms. Eileen's other underwear near her waistline, the friend said, "Look, Eileen, my body is larger than yours!"

"You're fat!"

"My rear end is so big, it wouldn't fit inside your tiny bloomers!"

And the steam started to build, threatening to erupt into a full-on screaming match. I knew I had to think on my feet and redirect the conversation. So, I convinced Ms. Eileen to make a pot of her favorite chicken soup with me. Tragedy averted, we sang to some Frank Sinatra music as we prepared our special lunch together.

As it happens, for some people, Alzheimer's can look like a loss of the client's verbal filters. This meant that I'd constantly be on damage control, trying to make up for whatever my client would bluntly say to others without being able to control her thoughts. Even then, I knew that this was my calling. There was something amazing about thinking up the right thing to say at the right time.

Work Expands

As I grew to love my job, I asked my manager, Maryann, to give me the grumpiest clients with dementia. It was rewarding to help them through their moods and watch them change while I was with them. I had several clients, all affected by Alzheimer's/dementia, and watching their improvement became almost addictive. It made my day when I made theirs.

Another Setback… Or Blessing?

By this time, it was 2005, and I was three years into the start of something wonderful. However, as God planned, I conceived my third baby: my beautiful Elizabeth. However, she had a rare heart defect: transposition of the great arteries (TGA). Because of this, she was extremely ill, so she needed me full-time. I put my career on hold once more because my kids were my first priority. And that is a decision I do not regret.

My Lizzy Loops grew up to be a mini-me. She's my youngest little angel, and I'm glad for every last thing I managed to do for her.

An Ode to My Mother

Throughout this turbulence, one person who stood by my side was my mother. Every bit Grandma's daughter, she was a hard worker who poured her lifeblood into raising me.

When I was a child with big dreams, she was my cheerleader and backbone.

When my path in life changed, she was right there to catch me when I fell.

When it came to making these sacrifices for my family, she was my inspiration.

She taught me how to work hard with her own example, and she supported me through sobbing sessions and downtimes, a calm, comforting presence that remained when everyone else I'd once depended on had left me.

Even now, at 79, she continues to see and support me through thick and thin. I couldn't be grateful enough for her support if I tried.

In a Nutshell: Finding My Feet

In the first decade of my marriage, I transitioned as I found myself again. I began as a comfortable housewife caring for her husband and kids, having given up on my passion. However, adversity and circumstances reminded me that I needed to be strong for my kids, pushing me back to my old passion of caring for the elderly. Unconventional as my journey was, I believe that it was beautiful just the way it happened, and I wouldn't trade what I learned from these years for a conventional degree. I was always where I needed to be, but it took me years of being lost to see that.

So yes, this period was riddled with questions and uncertainty, but it was essential to help me grow into a person whose cup was full enough to pour from. A person whose life was full enough of love and whose family was complete so that she'd be tethered to sanity and reality as she cared for others.

In Hindsight

Looking back, I believe that devoting the second phase of my life to my kids was one of the best things that could have happened to make me successful in caring for the elderly.

You see, when I saw that ad for a caretaker for the elderly, the skills I needed were those I learned from caring for my kids. I had the patience to answer the same questions until my mouth ran dry, and I had the superhuman power of a mother to juggle between different tasks, find the perfect distraction, and keep people occupied while I got my work done. I'd learned from dealing with my husband how to maneuver difficult people and from my kids how to love people who sometimes (okay, a lot of the time!) drove me up the wall with their antics.

Like I always say, you need to care for the old as you care for the young, and between Grandma and my kids, life taught me how to do both.

Chapter 3:
My Time with Mr. E

Some people come into our lives and leave imprints on our heart[s], and we are never the same. –Flavia Weedn

During the early years of my career, I battled with brief spells of purpose amidst life hurling me against the rocks every time I began to see the shore. I had precious few people who stayed with me and became my emotional backbone. Two such gems you've already met: Grandma and Mom. My beautiful daughters gave me the willpower to live for them. Amongst the six of us girls (Grandma's memory included), we were an unbreakable unit.

However, as I sought to expand my horizons, I'd need much more than family. I needed to see how all people (especially men) weren't like my father and husband. In short, I needed to form a bond with a man that I could respect and admire.

And such a man was Mr. E.

Meeting the Man Who Changed My Life

I stood outside a split-level house in Plainview, New York, my hand hovering above the doorbell as I checked my appearance one last time.

Nearby was a beautifully landscaped garden, decorated with lovely, neat shrubs with an obvious lack of flowers. I'd later find out that this was the work of Mr. E's brother-in-law Arnie. But for now, I was terribly new to the setting and wondering what it had in store for me. I took a deep breath and rang the bell. It was a momentous day in 2007 because I was finally returning to work part-time after two years. My Lizzy Loops was finally feeling a bit better, freeing me up somewhat. I just hoped the client wouldn't be too grumpy or give me too hard a time.

All I knew was the following:

- He lived in Brooklyn

- He was a Kosher Jewish man with Alzheimer's

- I wasn't supposed to bring any other food into his Kosher home.

- My main duty was to get him out of the house somehow. This sounded foreboding, because what sort of recluse would he be?

- My job included light housekeeping.

- I was supposed to be there every Saturday and Sunday, from 10-2.

I went over the list again, hoping and praying that I hadn't forgotten anything. On the other side of this door stood the man I'd be dealing with for years, perhaps. I *so* hoped he'd be nice!

As I stood in a puddle of anticipation and nervousness, the door squeaked slightly on its hinges. A man emerged. He was a tall man, around 5' 8", looking as if he weighed around 140-150 pounds. He wore framed glasses, a button-down shirt, and the pair of slacks I'd see him in every day. I wondered what his voice would be like. Friendly? Domineering? Grumpy? Petulant?

"Where have you been?"

I was taken aback for a moment. I'd never met the man before! But then the quick thinking I'd practiced with my kids and Ms. Eileen kicked in.

I replied, "I missed you, sir. I couldn't wait to come back!"

And just like that began a friendly banter that would be the hallmark of our conversations.

Breakthroughs

Right from the first day, I felt as if I was making headway with Mr. E. He was a pleasant man, and we spoke for hours as I tried to get a clearer picture of his life. Here's what I found out pretty much right away:

- He was born in December 1923.

- He had two wonderful children and three grandchildren that he loved dearly: two boys and one girl.

- He loved owls.

- The massive collection of artwork in his house was from the different countries he'd traveled to with his late wife Myra.

- He was quite easy to talk to because the conversation was taking hardly any effort from my side.

So far, so good!

But then we came to the one thing I *had* to do: get him out of the house. Once we were comfortable and acquainted, I asked him if we should go out. How hard could it be for a nice old man to go see some sunshine?

I was confident as I inquired, "Sir, would you like to go out?"

"*No!*"

It turns out, I was wrong. How wonderful!

I was speechless with surprise. This was so unexpected! I'd failed on my very first day! But I refused to give up so easily. For the present, however, while he was still disgruntled and defiant, I'd get to know him a bit more through conversation.

Rapport, as before, was comfortable and free. I watched his face light up as he spoke of his adorable redheaded granddaughter, giving me a hint of how he loved little children. So I tried again, more craftily this time as I took an indirect approach. I started with a question rather than a request, pulling out a picture of my baby Liz, who was just turning two.

"Mr. E, could you please help me pick up a present for my two-year-old daughter Elizabeth's birthday?"

He surprised me with a response as emphatic as the first. He jumped off the couch, exclaiming, "Of course I can, let me get my jacket!!"

That's when realization struck me: for a client with this horrible disease, "no" doesn't always mean a "no." For Mr. E, it was merely an automatic response he'd learned, perhaps as a toddler.

On another note, I also saw that Mr. E, like myself and countless others, needed to feel needed again. He'd lost all his adult responsibilities: his car, finances, and the ability to go out by himself. I realized that he wanted what so many others truly need from life: a purpose, a reason to get out of bed every morning. And that my job as an Alzheimer's caregiver was to give him one.

Down Memory Lane

As I got to know Mr. E better, we fell into a working camaraderie. Every weekend, I'd show up at his place to find him playing solitaire at his kitchen table or doing a jigsaw puzzle, both of them activities for one. Every time, I'd make progress encouraging him to leave the house more and engage in outdoor activities. We'd mostly go out for an adventure together when I was there, helping him see the beauty in interacting with others.

Other times, we sat in the comfort of his home, exchanging stories. I loved going down his past with him, forgetting all about my present as I was enthralled by the fantasies of a land that seemed so distant and yet so real. In these stories, I got to know Mr. E better and better as I simultaneously figured out how to help him.

The Innocence of Childhood

Mr. E was born in Brooklyn. Back then, his family did not have much money. His father was a painter, and his mother was an excellent cook. Every Friday after school, he'd walk into the apartment building where he lived and smelled the challah bread and roasted chicken. He'd inhale the aroma deeply, giving a satisfied "Mmmm, good!" as he looked forward to the delicious food awaiting him. As he recounted this memory,

Mr. E relived the smells and recreated the gesture. His doing it as a boy must have been adorable!

These happy memories, like most memories, had a bittersweet edge to them, too. Mr. E lived near lots of Italian families and enjoyed going to their homes. As I said earlier, our Italian community was centered around family and Catholicism, and Christmas united both. Seeing them, Mr. E recalled wishing that Santa would come to "this Jewish boy's house," but he never came.

Once, when Mr. E badly wanted a bicycle as a young boy, he secretly worked for the *Saturday Evening Post* magazine. Without telling his parents, he went and sold them at the city's subway station, working and pinching and scraping until, one fine day, to his surprise, he won a contest. And the prize was a beautiful bicycle with white-walled tires. Oh, did he *love* that bike! He cherished it like anything until, one day, he went upstairs to his apartment to use the bathroom. When he came down, he saw his beloved bike driving down the lane. Someone had stolen it. As a young and innocent boy, he ran after it, panting and puffing, shouting at the person to stop, but his tiny legs failed to catch up. He was devastated as, with a broken heart, he waved goodbye to his prized possession.

On a lighter note, Mr. E loved Nathan's Famous hot dogs. His father would take him there to eat as a child, but he'd tell Mr. E not to tell his mother. The implication, of course, was that the hot dogs were non-Kosher. Mr. E's laughter as he related this story was infectious, dispelling any negativity from other memories.

Teenage Mischief

When Mr. E got to college, tuition was free. "Free for me," he specifically said. He graduated with a degree in geology.

"Rocks, Mr. E?" I enquired in mock incredulity. "What were you thinking?"

"Rocks in my head," he chuckled.

What he did get out of college, I'd say, was more precious. It was priceless. He found his future wife. They were both sixteen, and she sat in front of him. Mr. E would be lost in nostalgia as he recalled those early days of their relationship. He'd poke her in the back with his pencil, watching her pretty, curly brown hair bobbing as she turned her tiny, petite frame around to face him. Myra was a cutie, as Mr. E put it.

Mr. E continued to torment Myra until she finally agreed to a date. This marked the official beginning of their young love that would blossom into so much more.

Once, Mr. E and Myra went on a date with friends at the amusement park at Coney Island in Brooklyn, the highlight of the place being the famous parachute jump. This 250-foot-tall steel structure wasn't for the faint-hearted. Waiting in line with Myra, Mr. E dared her to go first, claiming that she had more guts than he did. He recalled how, petite but determined, she'd taken the chance and gone first.

"I would never take the chance!" I laughed.

"Neither would I," he replied with the characteristic twinkle in his eye.

One Saturday, I took Mr. E to visit that park, and we relived that dare. We laughed hard at the story of how he'd teased Myra at the park, admiring her courage at the same time.

Army Life

After a few years of dating, Myra and Mr. E became extremely close. However, fate knocked on his door again, and Mr. E was drafted into the army in 1942. There was a poster from Uncle Sam that said "I want you," he recalled, pointing with his finger as he saw the poster in his mind's eye.

At this point, Myra wanted to marry him, but he refused. He didn't want to leave her a widow if he were killed, he told her. However, all the while he was away, he exchanged some heartwarming letters with her that his daughter still holds close to her heart.

After basic training, Mr. E was sent to Ohio for specialist training, but that was cut short. He was then shipped over and went to Marseilles (thankfully, not Normandy!), participating in the Battle of the Bulge.

After this battle, instead of coming home for furlough and then going to the Pacific, he pulled some strings to stay in post-war Germany for an extra year. He'd hoped it would be safer. He had no idea that Japan would surrender after Hiroshima and Nagasaki. Nevertheless, during army service, Mr. E was promoted to become a Master Sergeant. I still remember him pointing to his sleeve.

"Three stripes up, three stripes down," he'd say with pride.

After his enlisted service was up, Mr. E accidentally enlisted for an extra year. Boy, was he sorry! In the meantime, he kept assuring Myra that his heart and soul were still hers. As soon as he was done, he came right back to her, surprising her when she was still in *Shiva* (seven-day mourning) after losing her mother. He was wearing his dress uniform and standing to attention when the door opened.

He had come back.

Married Life

After he returned, Mr. E married his sweetheart in a small ceremony and started learning the carpet business as an apprentice. Soon, he'd found his feet with a carpet business of his own. By this point, Myra was a psychologist. Together, they were complete. He loved his wife so much that he went ahead and carpeted their entire home. I still smile as I remember him relating his bride's reaction:

"Carpet in the kitchen?" she exclaimed, "No one carpets the kitchen!"

She then proceeded to be mad at him for a good few minutes. Their home, as Mr. E laughed, was "distinctive" with the carpeting. Myra threatened to roll him up inside said carpet and toss him out of the door, Mr. E recalled, tears of laughter in his eyes as he guffawed uncontrollably.

To my surprise, the kitchen carpet stayed. It was there until one Seder (a customary Jewish meal) when Myra had the kitchen carpet shampooed. And that evening, during the Seder dinner, she dropped beef gravy on it. After that, she lost it so badly on the carpet (and the carpet man!) that the very next day, she chucked it out and had linoleum floors put in instead. She couldn't do much with the carpet man, though! Once again, Mr. E laughed as he recalled his wife's anger.

As a couple, Mr. E and Myra traveled a lot to Israel and France, both of which they loved and where they had friends to visit. He carried a heavy piece of artwork they believed was a figurehead of some sort—another of his eccentricities. He'd always complain to me about how heavy it was to carry, and given how much they traveled, it must have meant a lot to them! In some ways, I suppose it's the weird habits that stick around in the memory to be cherished, no matter how cumbersome they may have been in the past.

Listening to Mr. E reminisce about the old days was one of the highlights of our time together. His stories about his marriage were a balm to my own hurt feelings. I, too, had met my sweetheart at sixteen, but he'd turned out to be the wrong person. My mother and I had been wrong in our choices of men. Now, as a mother of three girls, it was a blessing to have found a man who had truly cherished his wife.

This story time was designed, of course, for Mr. E's benefit. I'd set time aside to listen to his Suitcase of Memories, as I call it, every visit. It deepened our bond, made him feel heard, and let me assess his memory and see how far it went.

At the end of every shift, I would ask Mr. E the same questions about his Suitcase of Memories to keep track of his memory:

"May I ask you some questions?"

"Of course!" was the reply.

"You married Myra?"

"Yes!"

"What did you study? Geology?

"Yes."

We'd then cover Geology having been a weird choice of degree, especially since he then went on to become a Master Sergeant and finally ended up as a "carpet man." Every time, we'd laugh at the absurdity of his journey.

Truth be told, Mr. E loved listening to his own story. Perhaps it was because listening to the story of his life in the past kept him grounded in the present. You see, it's terrifying to be losing your memories. As a caregiver, I made it my job to keep the memories safe and to keep Mr. E engaged. I'd do what I could so he wouldn't fear forgetting himself while I was there to remind him.

And that's what I'm doing to date: keeping my friend's memories alive and safe.

Gaining Momentum

Exchanging stories and having heart-to-hearts, our bond deepened until we were exchanging jokes. In his memory, I've compiled some of my best memories with him.

For the Love of Food

Mr. E loved the song "That's Amore." One of his favorite lines in it was,

"When the stars make you drool
Just like pasta e fasule, that's amore."

Of course, I wasn't letting him get away with that!

I asked, "Is pasta e fasule really amore?"

"*No way!*" was our joint reply.

For reference, pasta e fasule is basically pasta with beans. We both hated the stuff.

The trick, of course, was to keep him laughing and joking in high spirits to lift his mood as a lone widower with Alzheimer's. I would make such comments often to bring bittersweet stories alive with humor and to bring him back to the present. Here's a peek at what our conversations were like:

"Dark or white turkey meat?"

"White," he replied.

"Great! I like dark turkey meat. We can be friends, ha-ha."

"Milk or dark chocolate?" I asked.

"Milk."

"Good! I like dark."

When I told him I liked sour pickles (he loved half-sour pickles), I said, "Great! We can remain friends!"

He laughed like anything at that.

As an afterthought, I once said, "You know, we can't fight. You like the opposite things."

"No competition here!" he chuckled in response.

Such light-hearted banter was normal in our conversations as we went out for lunch almost every visit. We were like two peas in a pod. He loved pastrami on rye with half-sour pickles at Ben's Kosher Deli and National Hebrew hot dogs at another Kosher deli called Boomy's. He also loved French fries and Doc Brown's root beer soda. Often, we'd go to a nice, old-fashioned place called The Milleridge Inn in a nearby village. We'd have a cup of afternoon coffee there with the blueberry pie he loved. Every birthday, I'd treat him to his favorite Chinese restaurant, where he relished the chow mein. We could only have meat at these Kosher places, but we enjoyed our food together.

Eating habits helped Mr. E to keep up with old eating traditions and to form memory patterns, and we soon fell into a comfortable relationship revolving around familiar settings and friendly people.

Cars, Music, and Wordplay

During car rides, Mr. E loved listening to Frank Sinatra and Nat King Cole, and we'd sing together ever so loudly! I still remember seeing him smile out of the corner of my eye, admiring the fall foliage. The fall season was when we sang the most, relishing the weather and the scenery. Mr. E also loved to sing the following:

- Dean Martin's "Standing on the Corner Watching All the Girls Go By"

- Martin's "I Am Gonna Sit Right Down (and Write Myself a Letter)"

- Fats Waller's "Your Feet's Too Big"

- Artie Shaw's "Stardust"

- The Glen Miller band's swing music

With the instrumental music, Mr. E would tap his feet to the beat and say, "Oh, yeah!" It was wonderful to see him enjoy these small things.

Mr. E loved his vehicles. As a child, it had been his bike. Now, he'd pretend to pout and cry when he remembered his beloved Buick that broke right before I started working for him. He told me how he had waved goodbye to it as they towed it out of the shopping center, his expression almost comical with mock grief. To him, that car must have been a form of independence, and I understood the pain behind his light words. Thankfully, our going out together could help with this!

Another time, when I asked him whether he liked cats or dogs, he wittily replied,

"I like Mrs. Katz."

I didn't know a Mrs. Katz, so I'm assuming it was his way of saying he preferred women over cats. It was proof that he hadn't lost his touch with jollity and liveliness. He could never resist a chance for wordplay and wit, and I encouraged it. It could help keep his memory active to make these connections and to be playful, and that was what I wanted.

Making Light of the Dark and Serious

Spirits and spooks were another topic of humor for us. Mr. E lived near a funeral home where the porch light was always on, but we never saw any cars or funerals there.

"Do you think anyone is home?" I'd ask him.

"I'll give you five dollars if you ring the doorbell," he'd laugh.

"Will you double the money if anyone answers?" I'd reply.

Of course, we knew that the only people who lived there were the sleeping dead. I never had the courage to take the dare and get those five dollars.

As a Jewish man, Mr. E told me during Passover that he was the King of Matzah brei. There was little we didn't joke about, including the morbid and the borderline unhinged!

Between Mr. E's sense of humor and his love of food and life in general, I was able to steer him out of his reclusiveness, and we made our way out into sunshine and laughter, helping him find happiness despite his condition. Full of life and mischief to the end, Mr. E was a gem to be around.

Further Headway

Of course, as a caregiver, I was also testing Mr. E's memory as I went along.

Once, when we visited the Hotsville Ecology Site, an animal preserve where they kept injured owls, we saw all his favorite birds. On the way back, I asked him to recall where we'd just been. He looked puzzled. Then I took out a brochure and showed him one of the owls on it.

Instantly, he remembered, "Oh, yes! That owl was hit by a car."

Instantly, I knew two things:

- He could still read because it told the story of why the owl was living in the cage was there at the preserve.

- He could recall specific events when they were tied to things he loved.

You see, sometimes it's better to test people using out-of-the-box tests in a non-stressful environment instead of giving them dedicated memory tests. Moreover, I was able to tailor my next step based on this little test: Now that I figured that his memory could be helped by things he loved, I decided to bring more of those into his life.

I began with his love for children.

Now, bringing children to Mr. E's house was a big no-no because we were not insured for it at Home Instead. However, I knew that my Liz would be a delight for him to be around and that she wasn't the kind to wreck things. So, working with Mr. E's daughter Rae and her attorney, we had a contract made up to take all liability off Home Instead and had my boss approve it. Now, I could bring Liz to work.

My Liz loved Mr. E, and he loved her. He had a lovely circular opening between his kitchen and living room and Liz loved jogging through it, her little three-year-old self toddling around, bringing him joy. Wheeling her to places in strollers and shopping carts and loving Liz gave Mr. E another purpose in life. He felt needed and wanted and proud, and he was much better for it.

What really helped was a solution tailored to the client, and that only happens when you understand them thoroughly.

Great News

One snowy day, I took Mr. E to the gerontologist for a memory test. There was snow on the ground, he was wearing a hat, gloves, and a winter jacket, and it was freezing cold. Yet, about five minutes after we settled in, the doctor entered and asked him what season it was, and Mr. E could not remember. My heart sank. I knew his disease was progressing.

You might ask, "Where's the good news?"

It turned out that this highly recognized doctor *specializing* in Alzheimer's was surprised that his disease wasn't progressing faster. This was probably because of all the recreation, laughter, and mental stimulation he was getting.

You see, with a disease like Alzheimer's, you can hardly hope to stop the person from deteriorating. However, with care and attention, you can slow it down. And I'm honored to have helped Mr. E, a man I respected and loved working with, retain his memories for longer.

The Story of the Dinners

Once, in a similar test, I wanted to see if Mr. E was eating the dinners made for him because he couldn't remember if he was eating food properly. I had my suspicions because his pistachio ice cream box (he loved the stuff!) seemed suspiciously empty every time I went, so he might have been bingeing on it whenever he felt hungry.

Therefore, on the next visit, I brought Liz over and asked Mr. E if he could serve her lunch. I wanted to check if he still remembered how. Thankfully, he prepared a lovely lunch on his own. He even got her a glass of cold milk. This way, I knew that he could make a light meal like a sandwich so he wouldn't go hungry and he could use the microwave and stove so he could eat healthy, properly (re-)heated food.

This way, I was satisfied that Mr. E would be all right in the food department on the days I was off. I was glad.

In a Nutshell: My Time with Mr. E

Among all my clients, Mr. E might have been the one I bonded most with. Perhaps this was because I was in a vulnerable position myself and because he was a gentleman—perhaps the first one I'd known up close. Or perhaps it was just his contagious love for life. In either case, I suppose I needed him about as much as he needed me.

Moreover, I also took a great deal of courage, inspiration, and hope from Mr. E's loving, caring nature, making him a godsend at the time, especially as I was beginning to work while caring for a child with special needs.

In Hindsight

Working with Mr. E was a milestone in my professional knowledge because as I was thinking on my feet around him, I was devising and storing ways in which I could better serve other elderly clients. This added information was much needed in my trove of experience.

For example, I learned how to take indirect approaches to convince them to do something. I learned how to subtly give people easy tasks to give them a sense of purpose, and how to carry out indirect memory tests on them so that I could tailor their care plans. Perhaps most importantly, I learned how to use humor to lighten one's mood and to tone down sad or bittersweet memories. This way, I could keep their memories safe, remind them of their past, and help them out of their melancholy by putting a funny or light spin on sadder events.

In short, Mr. E was a crash course on caring for the elderly in different ways because all he needed was company and for me to think innovatively. What I learned from that innovation would come in handy throughout my career.

Chapter 4:
New Beginnings

Life is about change. Sometimes it's painful, sometimes it's beautiful, but most of the time it's both. –Kristin Kreuk as Lana Lang

Do you know the feeling when you're on a pirate ship ride at a carnival, and it gives you a few small swings as it gains momentum? When your body starts tensing up, and you take a deeper breath to stabilize yourself before your stomach starts threatening to spill its contents in public? Well, my life until 2008 was perhaps similar to these first few swings where there are lurches and jolts, but you aren't losing your mind. Such was my life when I was married and trying to maintain my relationship with Steven, simultaneously taking care of my work and kids. It wasn't really bliss; on the pirate ship, you know you'll get only one or two of those less-terrifying swings until you're screaming your lungs out. But the gentle swaying is, perhaps, what prepares you for the rough swings. 2009 was when these violent swings happened.

A Failing Marriage

They say that you need to let go of things you think are indispensable in the present so that you can make way for better things. For a long time, I'd been chasing stability, both financial and emotional, especially for my young children. 2009 was the year I stopped doing that and changed so radically that I'd never be the same again. It was painful because it meant accepting that the marriage that I'd been committed to for years was failing and that I'd have to leave the life I was now familiar with. However, it certainly led to something beautiful. It was a much-needed change that made way for wonderful beginnings.

Although my marriage with Steven had begun as a beautiful union where I thought we were completing each other, marriage was not the perfect team I'd imagined. Yes, in the beginning, it felt like he was the dream man with his financial stability making up for my failure to become a nurse. His need for a stay-at-home wife completed my aversion to all things career-oriented because I'd lost my chance at my dream career. My need to care for someone completed his need for someone to make his house a home.

When the charm of new beginnings started wearing off and Steven started controlling me, I tried to stay true to my vows and make the marriage work. By this time, I had my Jill, and I could not bear to leave and raise her fatherless. Heaven knows I had enough scars from being left by my father to want a complete home for my daughter. And then, as my daughters entered my life one by one, I'd decide to stick around longer to give them time with their father, hoping things would mend. But they didn't.

My restlessness and entrapment in the limits of my own house (not home!) continued to grow, but I couldn't leave. I was completely financially dependent on my husband, and, with little kids in the picture, I could not be rash. I needed to have a practical plan to support us. So when I saw that ad from Home Instead, it felt like hope. I took the job, met Mr. E, and saw what love was actually supposed to look like. I think that sealed the deal for my marriage.

Final Straws

As I said, leaving was still not a practical option because you need a *lot* of money to support a family of four, and I was still new at my job. It paid way too little to take this big step. However, one night, Steven took things too far. I knew, then, that I had to make the decision quickly.

It was a normal night, and I was volunteering as a 4th grade religion teacher. This was all part of my regular schedule, but then one student's mother arrived extremely late. Steven kept calling and harassing me, asking when I was going to return home because he had dinner ready. When I told him about the situation, he told me to just leave and come home. I knew I couldn't just leave the kid by themselves, so I put my foot down and stayed.

I suppose that was a sort of ultimatum from him because I came home to see the clothes and toys I'd kept for the poor scattered all over the driveway. My daughters were crying hysterically in the house. That night, he took away my cell phone, the house phone, the remote control, my car keys, and the computer keyboard.

At this point, I admit that I got too hurtful with my words and that we were toxic to each other together. Yes, he'd accommodated my work schedule and let me work and volunteer and study at the same time even though we'd initially planned on my handling the home front. Yes, he'd taken on making dinner and handling some of the chores while I was still not a breadwinner for the house. But yes, he'd also given me years of this behavior: anger, control, and harassment.

Working with Alzheimer's clients had taught me that it was possible I had not been able to respond to Steven's demands correctly. You see, when a client is being difficult or having a tantrum, you need to find out what is bothering them, get into their past and present, figure out their tics and what soothes them, and treat them accordingly. In our marriage, as with my work, it takes two to destroy a working relationship. I, too, needed to develop the skills necessary to create a well-balanced marriage, and I take ownership of that fact. I'm older and wiser now, and when I look back, I can admit to myself and others that I had a lot to learn.

But back then, Reader, I lost my mind. I knew I wanted to leave with my daughters right then because my daughters needed to see a happy marriage, even though I didn't have enough money to support the entire house.

In September 2009, our time together was finally over. It was time for the seeds of something new to be planted.

A Life of Separation

When Steven left, it was very different from when my father had abandoned me. However, because of that old trauma, I was expecting the separation to be horrible. You see, I'd spent my childhood hoping and wishing and praying that my father would come back to me, but when he returned years later, I was devastated to see him in his true colors. Perhaps I had always seen my father through the lens of an innocent, loving child but the second meeting confirmed the dreadful reality that he'd chosen drinking over our family. Yes, I had forgiven him long ago, and I loved him, but when I saw that history might repeat itself, I was afraid. What colors would Steven show me and our kids? How would I handle my kids' questions and their pain of separation? I had never remembered my father's bad side, after all.

At this point, I knew that my daughters would likely pine for their father, but I dreaded him returning and continuing his verbal abuse. The following years were awful. I stayed married to him, praying that he and

I could both try and that he would change his ways. For years, I tried to mend the relationship, but it was beyond repair. He was the same man, and I was mentally done with the marriage.

To Steven's credit, though, when I asked him to leave, he did, giving us a roof over our heads while I figured out the upkeep of the house on my own. He also helped pay for the girls' colleges, cars, and other expenses, so I had his support even though I could not build a marriage of love with him. In some ways, his continued support was an extra blessing because I knew that even if we separated ways, my daughters wouldn't be robbed of their father. I would be free to look for love elsewhere without hurting them irreversibly. With Steven, it wasn't abandonment for my kids: it was us choosing to separate so we could give them and ourselves some peace.

On the other hand, I was still working with Mr. E. I saw what a good marriage could look like when there was mutual respect and love from the man who had truly adored his bride. I wanted to enjoy my spouse wholeheartedly like Mr. E. Perhaps this was why I loved my work so much: it gave me a window into lives of love, so I knew what it looked like.

If separation was painful, it was made more so because I couldn't move on, and I didn't want to look back. The past was painful and the future was unpredictable. And in it all, I wondered what love would look like for me.

The Work Front

Three to four months before our separation, I finally graduated college in May 2009. Things were looking up for my budding career because now I wasn't the uneducated, lower-level worker anymore: a few more accreditations, and I could begin working professionally.

In December 2009, around three months after our separation, Home Instead got new owners. At first, I felt a great deal of apprehension because I wasn't sure what was to become of me. I desperately needed a promotion at work because I needed the money, but my new bosses didn't know the first thing about me! How would they know about my current clients and the way I dealt with them? The uncertainty was building up further.

However, the new ownership turned out to be a blessing in disguise. With our new bosses, the company started looking to expand its business and to find new clients. At this point, I realized what a gem Maryann (my manager) was: She suggested to them that they promote me to be their marketer. She knew that the company needed to reach more clients and that I was going through a separation with financial hardships, and she put me forward to meet our bosses.

Mark and Nicole Labib, my new employers, were a young, beautiful couple with two small children. They were extremely accommodating, and I liked them immediately. They gave me the gift of believing in me and the chance to try my hand at the position even though I was just a caregiver back then. Additionally, they gave me full rein to go crazy and be creative with how I wanted to promote their name in the industry. Perhaps more importantly, though, my new salary was much better than my previous one, helping me meet my family's needs.

Thus, in 2009, I became the face of Home Instead, my beloved workplace, as their Community Liaison. Under my new responsibilities, I was still working on the weekends with Mr. E and, during the week, I was putting in three full days at Home Instead's office. My career was looking up! I thank God that the position worked for me and that my prayers were answered.

On the other hand, my mother was taking care of my kids, quite like Grandma had taken care of me. Under her watchful eyes, they learned the power of empathy and the importance of family, getting the love and care they needed. Unlike Grandma, though, Mom stayed with them as long as they needed her and is still ever-ready to help them through a crisis as their beloved Nanny.

With my home and work life settled, I was able to focus on improving my skills as a dementia caregiver. To do this, I kept taking on as many courses and certificates as I could. This way, I could become an even more highly paid professional, as I'd have those certificates behind my name. I was reading and researching as much as I could, wanting to do my best to advance my career and to care for the elderly.

I was reaching some kind of stability, and I was extremely grateful for it.

In a Nutshell: The Year 2009

If life until 2008 was a slow-ish preparation for the violent swings of a pirate ship at its fastest, then 2009 put me on one of those scary corner seats and swung me a full 360 degrees, jolting me every time I tried to breathe.

The minute I thought I was finally done studying formally, I walked into a separation. While I was still reeling from my new reality, dealing with the cocktail of my emotions, Home Instead got sold. As I tried to process this with my exhausted brain, I got a much-needed promotion and had to adjust to the extra work *while* I dealt with Single-mom-ism and having to manage all the bills for the first time. I also had to learn to market the company, having never done anything of the sort.

Would life ever reach that near-equilibrium for a few short moments before the next lurch, or had my pirate ship suddenly become a yo-yo that someone was swinging in full circles, never to stop?

Only time would tell.

In Hindsight

As an Alzheimer's caregiver, I think this year was a skill-builder in terms of multitasking and keeping my personal and professional lives separate. You see, it's well and good to be an excellent caregiver when everything is hunky dory at home. The true test is whether you can keep your anger and frustration inside when you're dealing with a helpless, fragile client. I was juggling between these two worlds, and it was an extremely challenging and yet enriching experience to have so much on my plate.

2009 prepared me for years of service to come, teaching me how to keep a smile on my face even when things were going haywire inside because that is essential for a caregiver.

Chapter 5:
Farewell, Mr. E

We both know there has already been a passing,
one that has left a wake as that of a great ship
that disturbs the sea for miles either side
but leaves the water directly at its stern
strangely settled, turned, fresh
and somehow new,
like the first sea there ever was
or that ever will be. –Owen Sheers, "The Wake"

I still remember, as if it had all happened yesterday, the day my best friend left me. He'd been an inspiration, a backbone, and a support. He'd shown me that there could be love and beauty in marriage. He'd loved my kids, and we'd practically become family to each other. He'd reawakened my passion to explore the depths of senior people's memories and wisdom and to learn from them. He was at once a role model and a dear friend.

Earlier, I spoke of the day I met Mr. E. It was a milestone in my life because I'd found a stable job with a client that I could truly love, one who inspired me and who left me feeling invigorated with his jollity rather than depressed by his pains. However, this point in my timeline is about the day he passed, another landmark in my life: one that marks the day I felt alone again. In this chapter, I want to devote some time to a man who touched me so much; his leaving left a scar so deep that it's still raw. I want to honor him by putting down the rest of my memories of a man who changed my life.

Declining Health

Between 2007 and 2011, I had four beautiful years with Mr. E, caring for him and growing to respect and admire him as I learned about his past, his customs, habits, preferences, and his witty, humorous side. Most of all, perhaps, I loved his ability to love and cherish because he made me feel important to him. We were great friends, and I'd begun to look forward to our weekends together. Especially when my marriage failed, and I was alone, trying to balance my kids with my work life, Mr. E supported me and was there for me, deepening our bond to newer levels.

However, with his age in the late eighties and the horrible condition he had, I had to see that Mr. E's mental and physical health was failing by inches. Yes, recreation, activity, and laughter could slow the process, but you can't reverse time or prevent the inevitable. So I promised myself instead that I'd witness his life to the very end and stay by his side, even if it was almost unbearable to see this end approach.

As his physical condition worsened, Mr. E got a live-in aide from Home Instead: Cynthia. He had severe lung cancer, and in his last few weeks, our car rides would include Cynthia and his oxygen tank, as well. I'd sometimes have tears in my eyes that I'd blink away, almost like you wipe away the first few droplets from a drizzle before the rain gets too heavy and you have to stop and wait for it to pass. Now wasn't the time to cry; it was a time to cherish and remember. There would be time to mourn later.

The End Draws Near

I wasn't the only one who saw Mr. E's death approach. He and his family knew it, too. I think he was glad it was almost over, though. He'd become lonely and frail and was in pain. It would be cruel to ask him to stay.

A few weeks before his passing, I arrived to find Mr. E playing solitaire at the kitchen table, as usual. However, this time, he was whispering to himself. As I approached, I saw that he was actually whispering to Myra. He was telling her how much he loved her and how he missed her, recalling their life together. I was glad his Alzheimer's hadn't stolen those precious memories from him, much as I felt as if the waves of grief were too much to bear.

For his sake, I'd hold myself together until the end, at least when he was around.

Rae, Mr. E's daughter, also sensed that she'd be losing her father soon. A few days before his passing, she gave her entire Barbie collection to my Lizzy, who had loved the man and brought him joy. Lizzy loved those dolls, and we still have them. Perhaps they remind both of us of Mr. E and the wonderful times we had together. Perhaps Rae had meant for them to be such a reminder, making them more than just a passing gift.

With these bittersweet last memories where we were trying our best to be strong and grab whatever memories we could, it felt as if those last days passed in a blur. We were waiting for the moment and dreading it. We were stuck in limbo, as if time had stopped but was still ticking closer to the hour. Expressions of grief awaited. Grief itself had already taken hold of us.

Shiva

Mr. E passed away on September 22, 2011. His body was carried out of the house "feet first," as he'd requested. Fulfilling his last wishes and remembering him was all we could do as we entered the period of his shiva.

It was like Grandma had left me all over again, only I was much older and thought I processed my emotions differently. I thought I had been prepared for the moment by his long ailment. However, the devastation that hit me was both real and potent.

When Mr. E left the world, my daughters and I experienced our first shiva, blurring the boundaries between Catholicism and Judaism. Mr. E was a wonderful man, and I'd cherish his memories according to his culture. I loved the man who had passed; that was enough.

At his shiva, I recounted the memories that Mr. E had shared with me. It was a week to be celebrated with his family in his memory, after all. In sharing these moments with his family and these warm memories, I realized that a Catholic wake wasn't what I wanted when I passed. I wanted people to remember me well and to learn from the experiences of my life as I learned from Mr. E's. You see, with traditional Catholic wakes, your body is laid out for people to see one last time, where a shiva is more a celebration of life and how people remember the deceased. Although I remain Catholic, I don't want to be waked at my funeral. I'd rather have a nice church service with a one-day celebration of my life rather than my death, with lunch for family and friends as my death unites them around me one last time.

As an Alzheimer's caregiver and, more importantly, as Grandma's little protegee, I always looked beyond age, race, religion, and the effects of medical conditions. I tried to look beyond the outside, deep into who the person was. This ability to be non-judgmental, accepting, and non-discriminatory was a gift from God, instilled and honed throughout my childhood.

In His Memory

To date, whenever it's Christmas, Rae sends me a much-treasured owl or some sort of other gift as I recall her father, who had loved the birds. We kept in touch, united by our memories of this wonderful man.

As Rae told me, they celebrate Mr. E's Hebrew date of death: the Yahrzeit in Yiddish. This turns out to be the 23rd of *Elul*, less than a week before *Rosh Hashanah* (New Year on the Hebrew calendar). As a man of laughter and celebration, I think it's fitting that his death be remembered along with new beginnings. For me, especially, a new life had begun with his impact on my being.

Just like the calendar system, I also began reading up on the prophets and laws of Judaism, building on my curiosity to know more about everything. I think it's beautiful how, thirteen years later, the dates important to him are still important to me.

Mr. E lives on in my heart.

In a Nutshell: The Passing

Mr. E's passing left a lasting mark on my mind and heart: a gaping void that may have diminished but has never been removed. He was a wonderful friend and client, and he introduced me to a world of love and laughter when I needed it desperately. Even in death, he continued to inspire me as I used his love as a standard for my relationships with others.

To Mr. E: Wherever you are, you're sorely missed.

In Hindsight

Part of the challenge of being an Alzheimer's caregiver for the elderly is "till death do us part," as they say. This means watching my clients waste away, participating in their funerals, and mourning for them. Until this point, the two people I'd been devastated at losing were Grandma and Mr. E. Both had left me broken, but their love had made me a stronger, better person.

Therefore, in retrospect, I believe it's worth the pain of separation if I get to share the beauty of my clients' last moments when they need support. In fact, losing such close elderly people may have prepared me and taught me to cherish my clients to the fullest before I lost them, and this became another principle of my practice: to be open to love deeply and to feel honestly and openly, even if the separation will come.

Yes, clients aren't family. But that doesn't mean they shouldn't be treated like family.

Chapter 6:
The Owl and the Promise

Death leaves a heartache no one can heal, love leaves a memory no one can steal. –Richard Puz

By the time Mr. E passed away, I had begun to get established in the Alzheimer's care department at Home Instead. Life was moving on, but the heartache from losing my best friend would not leave me. I was trying to love my new clients almost desperately as I tried to help families make the most of their loved ones' last days. I found comfort and solace in seeing other elderly Alzheimer's clients feel better under my care. However, sometimes, especially on days that had once been important to Mr. E, it got a little overwhelming. But even then, I believe the memory of love is more healing than the crushing pressure of grief.

This chapter is about one of those days.

Wherein I Try (and Fail) to Move On

As the clients rolled in, I tried to keep myself busy caring for them and earning a living for my own family. I was promoted at work (a story for another day!) and had to deal with Home Instead's marketing, reputation, and quality assurance. I was also going to be promoted to work as a trainer for Home Instead caregivers now, so that was another role I had to fill. Simultaneously, I was trying to work on my accreditation and deal with other Home Instead clients. In my whirlwind of a schedule, I was able to distract myself from the memory of Mr. E's passing. At least, I was mostly able to function properly.

One fine day, I was driving to a quality assurance visit, seeing to a Home Instead caregiver's client, Marie. Marie had recently fallen out of bed and broken her hip during the evening hours when there was no aide to care for her, and her family had requested Home Instead to provide an aide to give care and support to her.

When I arrived, Marie was inconsolable. She was crying and asking for her mother, desperately wanting to join her mama in heaven. She had Alzheimer's, too, which didn't help matters because without having worked with her long-term, I didn't know what worked to comfort and pacify her. My primary job was to convince her to do her physical therapy, but it was an ordeal trying to calm her down in the first place. How do you calm someone in pain, desperate for a loved one they can't meet, being forced into an activity that will drag them closer to a life they don't want?

Marie passed away that evening. And with her, the stranglehold I'd had over my emotions since Mr. E's death broke. Marie's desperation reminded me of Mr. E's last days, sitting at his kitchen table alone and whispering to Myra as his lung cancer kept him in incessant pain. He'd been desperate too, and it broke my heart to see the raw emotions on display. Mr. E, a jolly man as he was, had never struggled so hard, but I was reminded of what his internal state might have been. It broke something inside me.

On top of everything, I'd been aware all day that it was Mr. E's birthday: December 19, 2011. It was not three months since he'd passed, and now, on his first birthday since he left us, the pain was still fresh. I'd just been holding it at bay as I continued with work as usual, but now I broke down completely. I missed my friend so desperately that I started praying and whispering "Happy birthday" to him between sobs. Since he'd always loved owls, I promised him I'd buy myself an owl necklace for Christmas in his memory.

Marie's death and her family's grief reminded me of Mr. E's death and my own grief. I wondered how long it would take me to recover.

A Memory of Love That No One Can Steal

Days passed since I'd last broken down after Mr. E's death. Life went on, and work continued. Marie was replaced by other clients as different Home Instead aides would ask for tips and assistance, and I kept training them. But even as things returned to normal, I remembered my promise to my friend: that I would go and buy myself that owl necklace for Christmas.

Christmas approached, bringing with it pre-Christmas parties and presents. Thus, on December 23, four days after my episode, I arrived at an office Christmas party to find Maryann standing by my desk. She had a little gift box in her hand wrapped in silver, and she looked puzzled.

"This is a very odd gift to give someone," she began. "I put it down three times, but something pushed me to buy this for you."

My curiosity grew at her strange words, and I wondered as I unwrapped the little box. And then, as I caught my first glimpse of what was inside, I gasped, and tiny pricks of tears formed in my eyes as they began to blur. There it was, my owl necklace. I hadn't told Maryann I wanted one, but here it was. Tears streamed down my face as I recounted my wish, and Maryann cried with me as she pulled out the receipt.

On it was the date she had purchased the gift: December 19, 2011. My friend's birthday.

The Promise

When I was gifted the owl I'd promised I'd buy, it was a momentous occasion and I wanted to mark it with a pledge to myself and my late friend. I meant to keep it as long as the owl and its memory stayed with me.

"For I know the plans I have for you," declares the Lord, "plans to prosper you and not to harm you, plans to give you hope and a future (Jeremiah 29:11, n.d.).

So, when I received my owl necklace, I made a promise to myself, the good Lord, and to Mr. E's memory: I would devote my life to helping those with Alzheimer's and dementia. The wish I'd made with Grandma over that bone a year before she'd passed away found a more defined renewal after I lost Mr. E. I knew my calling, and I wanted to immerse myself in it fully.

I believe that God breathes a calling into babies' souls. Sometimes, it takes a few falls in life to see these wonderful gifts, and I had found mine at this point. I felt as if my life was predestined to work with the elderly, especially those who need hope at the last of their lives. My promise was to honor this calling.

In a Nutshell: My Calling, Renewed

Although losing Mr. E was a major blow in my life, I believe the true beauty in his passing was that I got to see him in his jolly, happy days and knew that he cared for me. Yes, his death was hard, but his memory was strong enough to motivate me when the going was rough. It gave me renewed determination to fight for my dream and passion.

In Hindsight

The gift of Mr. E's memory and the promise I made to him had a profound effect on my professional life because I continued working with renewed zeal. I was determined to do my best because the owl on my neck reminded me that this was my calling.

You see, success in a field as demanding as caring for the elderly has more to do with a driving force than an old passion. Yes, it was my childhood dream, but my driving force became the constant reminder that this is who I was meant to be. As long as I knew that, I could pour heart, soul, and lifeblood into caregiving and training others to give quality care. This became what marks my work as a professional helping clients with dementia and Alzheimer's.

Chapter 1:
The Start of Something Beautiful

It's true that we don't know what we've got until we lose it, but it's also true that we don't know what we've been missing until it arrives. –Unknown

Do you know the feeling when the pirate ship ride slows down, swaying gently before it stops? When your stomach stops churning and you take in deep gulps of fresh air to soothe your exhausted body? Yes, you get on the ship on purpose. Yes, there are tears of joy in the ride as well as screams of fear (for those who aren't as brave as Myra, with her parachute jump, at least!), but when the ride ends at long last, all you want is the peace and stability of solid, firm ground under you.

The pirate ship of my life finally began to slow down as I found what I'd been seeking for for decades. It happened when I met the man who brought me joy when we promised to stick to one another, and when we joined hands to begin a new leg of our journey side by side, hand in hand, experiencing life through the lens of love.

It happened when I met Bobby, the love of my life.

Hopes and Prayers

After Mr. E left me, I was determined to live life to the fullest, just as I had promised him that I would respond to my calling as a caregiver to the elderly. Mr. E's presence, while it lasted in my life, was one of quiet comfort and support. He was there behind me, his stories ready to transport me into the world of love and laughter that he had shared with his beloved wife Myra. Now, I was determined to live life like he did: with love and merriment.

So when, at the end of 2009, I could see an end to my financial crises, I looked inward at my family. It was fairly full, with my daughters growing up, and the five of us (including Mom) having a strong bond. I was now a trainer at Home Instead, so my salary was good, and I didn't have to do too many home calls anymore; I just went when I was needed for an expert opinion and pointers. However, I felt that we were missing the male father figure—the one I hadn't had past the age of five, either. Probably because she was missing this figure and troubled by my fights with Steven, my Jill got pregnant as a very young teen and had Natalie. I knew that she needed a full family to feel loved and complete. I had seen my brother suffer when my father had left, and now I didn't want Jill, Kim, and Lizzy to suffer and break away from our family. Moreover, I also desperately wanted a man who would love me, who I could be vulnerable around without him taking it as an invitation to control me.

At this point, I was still married to Steven. However, when I compared him to Mr. E, I felt as if our relationship could not work. Steven wouldn't change, and I did not have the emotional or mental capacity to be in a loveless marriage any more. I wanted to start over, back from the beginning where the negative memories wouldn't haunt me. And so, we got divorced. The year was 2012, and the divorce was final. There was no more looking back; I just had to charge forward.

And so, I started my prayers, asking the Good Lord for a *Beshert:* a soul mate sent by God. I will admit that I was strangely specific about the man I asked God for. A tall man who would be caring and who would love making a woman laugh. He had to be an outdoorsman, looking for an old soul, and marriage-minded. On top of everything, I wanted to share a marriage like Mr. E's and Myra's with my future husband.

If only my family could be complete, I'd be contented.

The Seeds of Love

In 2013, the year after I broke the knot with Steven, I met Bobby. He was 6'1", weighed 200 pounds, had blue eyes, and was mild-mannered and kind (strangely specific, right?). He'd send me inspirational quotes every day, one of which is heading this chapter. This means we also had regular correspondence to cherish all our lives and then leave behind, just like Myra and Mr. E's letters!

Had I found Bobby, or was he sent from above? I don't know. All I know is, as you can expect, I fell head over heels for him right away.

On our first date, Bobby and I met at the Milleridge Inn in the village where I used to take Mr. E. I unburdened my heart to him, telling him all about the friend I'd lost and how much I missed him. It was liberating to speak to someone so openly and for him to listen to me, adult to adult, without showing judgment! We fell into easy conversation, and soon we'd decided to continue the relationship that had begun to form between us.

Over six years, Bobby and I got to know each other and got acquainted with each other's kids. Bobby had two kids: Ryan and Brooke. Just as Jill had suffered from my failing marriage with Steven, Brooke and Ryan had also suffered terribly when Bobby's marriage fell apart. We both needed a stable blended home for our children's sakes, if not our own. Spending time together, our relationship grew stronger, and I knew that he was the man I could trust with my life: the man I'd love to wake up to in the morning and share my heart with in the evening.

Wedding Bells

Reader, I married him. But this time, it was not a marriage of mutual need and desperation as it had been with Steven, where he was the alternate to the career I could not have. With Bobby, I was walking into the marriage independently, knowing him and having thought out my decision thoroughly. We were getting married to build our family together and to be each other's company and emotional support and not for other pressures or expectations.

My "Big Doggy," as I call my husband, once said, "I'm going to make many of your days."

He *would* make my day ever so many times, and I would make his. It was as if we were meant to be together all along, and that everything in life up to this point was preparing us for our lives together.

On October 7, 2018, in a lovely barn overlooking a lake in Pennsylvania, we exchanged our vows together with our five children, friends, and family. Our wedding song was "God Blessed the Broken Road" by Rascal Flatts, which beautifully describes the bumpy paths that led us to each other (remember I asked for a marriage-minded outdoorsman? He's both!) Through all these trials, tribulations, and heartbreaks, I would not do things differently. My wedding day was the day I felt my life was full.

On the other hand, Steven also married a woman who loved him, who he could love in return. As we went our separate ways and embraced this new stage in our lives, we forgave each other and became better people for all the mistakes we had made, resolving that we'd do better in our second marriages. We're still in contact, and he spends time with our daughters, so they're lucky to have two fathers who care about them so much.

In a Nutshell: Marriage and Settlement

Marriage with Bobby was like the beginning of my Happily Ever After. At the end of the day, I realized that it's not necessary that our past traumas resurface in our lives. With hope, patience, and prayer, we ended up finding our purpose and contentment in life. All it takes is to accept our trials peacefully, knowing that we need to grow into the role that will bring us joy.

Previously, I often had to force-convince myself that my glass was half full. Now, it was overflowing with the love and laughter of our household. Such was the effect of meeting and pledging myself to Bobby, my better half.

In Hindsight

Although life threw many lemons at me, I believe that each one prepared me to deal with people who had their own share of lemons hurled at them. You see, while people like Mr. E gave me a window into what love could look like, there were so many others who didn't have the smallest taste of it. Life taught me how to understand the pain of others while it prepared me for my own happiness, so I'm grateful for the trials just as

I'm grateful for the wonderful man I found to complete me. Accepting this and finding my peace makes me a much better practitioner because when you're at peace and your cup is full, you can pour an endless stream of joy and encouragement into others.

Chapter 8:
Looking Ahead

Upon the edge of time, we stand,
With dreams and hopes at our command,
A future vast, with skies so wide,
Where possibilities reside.
The past is but a shadow cast,
A memory that fades so fast,
But in our hearts, a light remains,
A hope that breaks through all constraints.
Through trials faced and battles won,
We move towards the rising sun,
With hope our guide, we journey far,
To find our place among the stars. –Langston K.

Everything I have related thus far was based on my memories of my turbulent past and how it changed me. It was about the battles I faced and the ones I won. It was also about the trials I went through that made me who I am today. On top of it all, it's about the hopes and dreams that sustained me as I got to where I am today.

Now, you might be wondering: Where am I today? Reader, I'm exactly where I wanted to be and where I'm meant to be. You see, our dreams are some of the first building blocks of our lives. Stick to that dream and persevere, and there's a high chance that you'll aim for the sun and end up in the stars, even if you have a couple (or couple thousand) asteroids hitting you on the way. And although my dream for progress continues, I am exactly where I need to be in my journey.

Life Continues: Gaining Further Expertise

After my second marriage, I think the pirate ship ride was over. In 2019, I became a Certified Dementia Practitioner (CDP) and a Certified Alzheimer's Disease and Dementia Care Trainer (CADDCT). I kept educating our Home Instead caregivers, giving seminars, and offering training programs to others in the geriatric industry.

In short, I continued to devote my life to caring for Alzheimer's clients and still do, though now as a certified trainer. It's heartwarming to find their voices, even if they've been reduced to simple, non-verbal responses like smiles or chuckles because every expression of happiness is a precious moment to be cherished.

Today, I'm working on starting my own business, all while I write seminars on dementia-specific care techniques, which I'll be covering in greater detail in a later book. For these training sessions, my daughter Kim helps me out, and we share our expertise together.

Volunteer Work Continues

Along with my professional work with the elderly, you can also find me hosting Alzheimer's/dementia support groups for families needing help in local libraries. Similarly, I'm running a crocheting group called "Seniors Helping Soldiers," making blankets and other things to donate to those in nursing homes or to homeless vets. All of this began when I had homebound seniors affected by Alzheimer's.

With all the work that pays in money, I feel that one should have a side engagement that brings pure, unconditional joy without asking for monetary returns. It's how I try to repay my debt to the community for all the good people in it who supported me. As Mr. E would say, it's a good Mitzvah.

Plans for the Future: Aiming for the Stars

Staying in the Loop

As I said, each client has to be cared for based on their individual needs, circumstances, and effects of their dementia. Each care routine must be person-centered, and to develop these routines, you need guidelines. For this, you need an experienced professional who works in the field and who knows exactly what problems other caregivers are likely to face. Such a professional has to have worked with people of different backgrounds and personality types, with different histories and progress notes with dementia. Therefore, my primary goal is to keep providing geriatric care as I develop unique training techniques in the industry.

While hands-on experience is great for developing my own techniques, I also believe in learning from others and their ideas. The more perspectives we have on this nasty disease and how to make it more bearable for clients, the better! When I learn about these techniques, I can try them out and see which ones work and which ones I can develop further to add to my repertoire. My goal here is to keep researching and staying in the loop so that my clients can have the best care I can give them.

Passing the Torch

What cues do you look for?

How do you balance hints from the client's past and present?

When do you call in the family, when do you need a therapist, and when should you use medication?

These and many more questions need experience to answer. In retrospect, I may have been better trained to deal with new situations with clients if I had a mentor to ask for help because, with split-second decisions, you need to take the right step quickly. To help with this, one of my most important roles at Home Instead is to be a trainer for new or less experienced recruits, being their go-to person in times of crisis.

My Own Startup: Empowering Professionals in Dementia Care

With experience as a caregiver and now as a trainer, I'm also working on a consultative platform that will help guide families of clients and will direct caregivers, even the ones outside of Home Instead. The platform will act as a place for people to ask me for help when they need an opinion about a care plan or help with a difficult client or family member. The logo for my business is an owl in memory of my late friend Mr. E, so send me a Harry Potter-themed letter (or email, or text–we're Muggles!) on my little owl if you need help.

My platform will do the following:

- It will give out-of-the-box strategies to deal with loved ones' behavior.

- It will give innovative ideas to get clients out of bed and ready for recreational activities.

- It will have guidance on how to integrate their Suitcase of Memories into their care routines.

- It will have tips on how to incorporate laughter and humor to lighten the mood as caregivers deal with the client and their declining memories.

- It will include things that I have learned and continue to learn from research and continued experience.

Seminars

Apart from my platform for advice, I also keep hosting sessions to give generic but innovative tips to other professionals in the field. After all, when I've spent so long learning these techniques, I believe I should pass on the basic skills to all. Here are the subjects for some seminars that I've recently hosted:

- bathing techniques

- building laughter and humor

- recreation and engagement

- why are Mom and Dad saying "no"?

- unraveling the individual again

- the independence approach

- finding purpose when purpose seems lost

- tricks to taking medications

- making memories from mealtimes

As a personal care attendant and former caregiver/companion, I love to share my experience with others entering the industry so that they can build on the techniques I have developed over a full career of service with Alzheimer's and dementia. I'm at the point where I'm experienced enough to share, and I'm getting ready to pass my knowledge on to the next generation as I prepare to take the back seat where I overlook and advise others. I believe it's the natural course of my career.

In short, my plans for the future are to keep learning and applying my skills as I begin to share them and pass them on to others.

In a Nutshell: Settling Down

With life slowing down and coming to some semblance of stability, I now have time to reflect upon my past and to think clearly about the future. Work is going well and marriage life is suiting me as I feel close to finding contentment in life. My kids are entering their independent lives, too. All is well until the next adventure life throws at us.

And when it does, just as in everything else, I have my hopes in God that all will continue to be well.

In the meantime, I fondly remember the journey that led me here, every step a rung on the ladder that led me to the rising sun of hope fulfilled and dreams promised. As Ayelet Waldman once said, "Memories, like dreams, are tools for understanding life…they provide an entry into the heart of what we have once experienced and help us make sense out of it after the fact" (Munshi, 2024).

From dreams to memories, I consider myself contented.

In Hindsight

Have you ever sat next to a calm stretch of still water, staring at your reflection, and felt a deep sense of calm? Ever looked out for that level-headed coworker to help sort out the mess of your thoughts or hear out your rants because talking to them calms you down? As with other things, I believe the positive energy of contentment is also contagious. If I as a caregiver am contented, I can incite similar feelings in others.

Perhaps it's good to look at it this way: You are like a mirror. If you're agitated deep down, that energy will affect your client and everything can come tumbling right down. However, if you're calm and in control, then you can deal with things clearly.

At this stage in life, clarity and calmness help me analyze my past and present and develop those caregiving strategies with care, aiming to pass on as much as I can.

Chapter 9:
The Joys of a Life Well Lived

A life well lived is a precious gift
Of hope and strength and grace,
It's filled with moments, sweet and sad
With smiles and sometimes tears,
With friendships formed and good times shared
And laughter through the years.
A life well lived is a legacy
Of joy and pride and pleasure,
A living, lasting memory
Our grateful hearts will treasure.
  –Author Unknown

As I near stability in my life, I look back at the times I've spent with gratitude. I remember the good times and the happy memories they left, and the difficult ones with the lessons they taught me. Through both, I cherish the people who stood by my side as family, friends, and coworkers, all enabling and supporting me to do the best I could as a professional caregiver.

With all that I had going for me, I'd like to devote a chapter to gratitude for the life God gifted to me and for the good I was able to do for the clients I worked with.

Realizations

Who would have thought that a Christian woman in her thirties could build a lasting relationship with an 84-year-old Jewish man diagnosed with Alzheimer's? But Mr. E and I did form a close relationship with our different worlds uniting to form something beautiful. And in my worldview tainted by anger and hatred, I realized that although we may all look different and believe in different things, at the core, we all need to feel needed and long for purpose and love. Once I learned to make this the basis of my worldview, my judgmental perspective on others took a U-turn as I tried to understand them with an open heart and mind. After all, if a religious Catholic woman's bestie is a Jew, we can't be all that different, can we?

In the book of Colossians in the bible, you see the words, "Therefore, as God's chosen people, holy and dearly loved, clothe yourselves with compassion, kindness, humility, gentleness and patience" (Colossians 3:12, n.d.). Similarly, in the book of Hebrews, you read, "And do not forget to do good and to share with others, for with such sacrifices God is pleased" (Hebrews 13:16, n.d.). With these Biblical texts, I combined my newfound knowledge of Jewish *Mitzvahs* (good deeds). Combining Christian teachings with my promise to Mr. E that I would perform *Mitzvahs* for others in his memory, I had enough to drive me toward good deeds toward the elderly and others. I think the joint teachings come together amazingly!

For the realization that I could have the best of both these worlds and that I could coexist and cooperate with people across ages, races, and religions, I am utterly grateful.

The Cup Is Always Half Full

Although I had long periods of uncertainty, listlessness, grief, and abandonment, when I look back at my life, I smile at how naïve I once was. In all those times of questioning what Fate had in store for me, I often lost sight of all that I was learning.

Losing Grandma and being left by my father, I learned to stand up for others who were grieving or abandoned, sticking to my dream of caring for the old and lonely.

Losing the hope of becoming a nurse, I got married and had my lovely children who I absolutely couldn't do without.

Stuck in a loveless marriage, I learned empathy for clients with rough marital lives or ones missing people who would cherish them.

Motherhood taught me patience and resourcefulness when dealing with the elderly.

As a single mother, I learned to appreciate my coworkers and friends and found out where my real support system lay.

Grieving for Mr. E, I made a strong promise that kept me going through rough days at work.

Financial instability showed me the materialistic riffraff I'd rather avoid now that I'm making more money.

Imagine, for a minute, that I wasn't born without my left hand. That I was blessed with both and had gone off to a normal college and become a mainstream nurse, working my way up through the regular ranks, and spending my entire life at the beck and call of senior doctors. Reader, I'd rather not.

Every three seconds, they say, a child is born. Each child comes with their own set of gifts and drawbacks. I believe that what the Lord didn't see fit to give me in the form of a perfectly normal body, he gave me in the form of compassion for my geriatric friends. With my unconventional path into my beloved career, I had the chance to explore different sides of life. I went through enough to build more empathy and was blessed with a unique path that continues to flourish with God's goodness and direction.

In short, every time I was down in the dumps, I was learning something or being guided toward greater things, and I could not be more grateful for the bumps in my life that launched me higher. Sometimes, you need those difficult situations to find your true purpose and the path that God intends for you.

Family: A Blessing Not to be Underestimated

When the going gets rough, you need a shoulder to cry on, a loved one to live for, and a friend to escape to. Throughout my personal and professional life, I was blessed with all three.

Grandma and Her Friends: My First Experiences

Although there is already an ode to Grandma right where my story begins, I suppose that any chapter about blessings in my life would be incomplete without mentioning her and her friends. They gave me love and friendship when Mom was struggling to earn and my father had left. I learned empathy as I spent time with their experience and wisdom and cared for them. With Gertie, I first experienced the devastating effects of Alzheimer's before I learned how to help others battle it.

Later in life, I'd draw on memories of these beloved ladies and my relationship with them when I cared for and tried to understand elderly clients I did not know.

For the love, understanding, and experience I got from Grandma's friends, I am honored to be a part of their Suitcases of Memories.

My Mother, My Cheerleader

Mom was one of my biggest supports while I grew up, believing in my ability to become a nurse despite my missing hand. When my father left, she took on the role of both parents and tried to do her best for Michael and me. When I faced setbacks in life and couldn't follow my passion, she propped me up and helped me land on my feet, being a shoulder to cry on and a hand that lifted me up. Her hard work in raising me inspired me to get up, dust myself off, and face the world as I fended for my kids as a single mother. Through those struggles, too, she cared for my kids, teaching them and giving them the time I couldn't spare from my busy schedule earning our living.

Mom is especially close to my Lizzy, and they've written a book together called *Teatime with Nana*. It's about a grandmother, Nana, and her beloved granddaughter Elizabeth, who loves visiting for tea and sleepovers. When Nana is diagnosed with Alzheimer's, Liz has to switch roles with her and host their tea parties. The book is designed to raise awareness in children and to show them how it's their responsibility to care for their grandparents in return when the roles are naturally reversed. Much the same way, my mother taught me a great deal of what I know about empathy and caregiving, and I have her to thank for my success as an Alzheimer's caregiver.

To date, Mom is called "Nanny" by all my kids and is absolutely adored by them. At 79, she's still the glue of our family and a huge supporter of my expanding career. The best is yet to come!

Danielle: My Childhood Friend

Yes, this section was supposed to be about family. But when you've been friends with someone for half a century, they become like family, too. Danielle supported me and encouraged me throughout my life, beginning after the devastating loss of Grandma, being a rare friend from my childhood when most people in my company were elderly. Even after 50 years of being there for each other, our friendship stays strong.

Danielle was a ray of stability and sunshine when the path was dark and uncertain.

My Big Brother: Together in Pain

Michael was a constant presence in my childhood, and I always knew that he had my back. I used to lovingly call him "Moon," almost as if he were a bright beacon in the darkness of night. Where I looked to Grandma for support, Michael suffered terribly from our father's abandonment. I suppose he also took it harder because he was older and had had more time with our father. Plus, as a young boy, he needed a male role model to guide him through life, and that was missing. Michael, Mom, and I used to go fishing together when we could. He was a great fisherman, although Mom and I were just okay.

I sometimes miss those good old days when we were young and innocent together. To date, we see each other every weekend, and my girls adore their "Uncle Moon," just as he dotes on them. I'm proud of all he accomplished in life, and I'm extremely grateful for his presence.

My Kids: The Light of My Eyes

When I was married to Steven and things were going south, I found solace and the strength to continue and honor my marriage vows when I looked at my kids. Honestly, I think I may well have given up on life and been unable to fight through those tough early days without them as my reason to wake up and their innocent love to fuel me through the hardest of times. Their existence motivated me to be the best Alzheimer's companion/trainer I could be.

Yes, I regret having been absent for a lot of their childhoods as I worked to support them, but they're the pride of my life. With their encouragement and their willingness to fend for themselves and cooperate, I had the strength to deal with the world outside. My kids appreciated me as they lived without complaint, knowing that I was working hard. For that, I'm utterly grateful.

As a little girl, my Liz would make and sell bracelets to support the Alzheimer's Association and The Alzheimer's Disease Resource Center in Long Island. She also worked on *Teatime with Nana* with my mother, as I mentioned earlier. Liz was a huge support when I cared for clients like Mr. E who enjoyed her company.

Today, my blended family with Bobby consists of five kids:

Jillian had a rough start with my failing marriage with her father, getting pregnant, and having a child when she was a young teen. However, she thankfully settled down and found success in her work life. Today, Jillian is 28 and is managing a team at a company that examines medical billing and finds the necessary codes to form bills correctly. I couldn't be prouder of her accomplishments as she continues to flourish.

Brooke is 26 and a teacher. Her love for teaching and caring for her little wards is incredible, and her heart and passion for her classroom is evident.

Ryan is 24 and a welder. The poor thing is the only boy among so many girls, but he found his feet in life, too!

From the age of just four, Kim began caring for Liz with her TGA. Here, she found that nursing was her calling. At 18, Kim joined Home Instead as a companion with me and her clients had wonderful things to say about her. However, she then moved on and today she works at an acute rehabilitation care center, caring for stroke and TBI patients. You can also see Kim hosting Alzheimer's training programs with me when I'm invited to host such a program. As a team, we help other care professionals better understand the tools and techniques I've used and discovered to deal with dementia. Now, Kim is 23 and has completed her Bachelor of Science and Nursing degree. She's a registered nurse.

Elizabeth is a college student at 19.

Our grandchildren are Natalie, Noah Peter (he passed away), Anthony, and Liliana. I love them dearly.

Watching all our kids on their way to standing on their feet independently makes my heart swell with pride to see them getting settled in their lives.

Bobby: My Soul Mate

Having seen my mother being abandoned by my father and losing my own marriage despite trying to maintain it, I'd settled for just looking at the storybook Happily Ever Afters like Mr. E's marriage from a safe distance. I never thought I could be loved that way. And then, when Bobby walked into my life, it was as if the picture was complete and my family was whole. With my "Big Doggy" by my side in a healthy marriage, my heart was overflowing with love and contentment.

What more can one wish for?

Mr. E: My Best Friend

As the client who supported me and became an invaluable companion who taught me about love and laughter, Mr. E made my life so much better as I laughed and ate with him and shared stories. I saw how beautiful his marriage was with both of them completing each other and having their separate, successful careers. They traveled together, had well-rounded kids, and lived for each other's happiness in their long lives together. It was like the movie *The Notebook*, and it truly inspired me.

The joy of a life well lived, as far as I'm concerned, is about having a successful marriage, family, and career that you love. It's about those priceless, raw things that money can't buy. Even after he passed, the memory of Mr. E's love kept me motivated for much longer as I strived to build a life like his. I'm blessed for all the ways my best friend and role model touched my life and my heart.

For Bosses and Workplaces

Maryann: My Workplace Backbone

Maryann has been a rock I leaned on at work. She supported me as I struggled with the early days of single motherhood, recommended that I should be promoted by Home Instead's new owners, and believed in me as she helped me find my feet. On top of that, she shared my pain and cried with me when I recounted the tale of Mr. E's owl and gave me strength because I knew I was not alone.

To anyone out there struggling, if you have one friend to cry with you, consider yourself lucky. I do.

Mark and Nicole: The Open-Minded Bosses

At Home Instead, I felt as if the people were like family. When you deal with grief and grim realities while working with aged people with deteriorating mental and physical health, it creates a sort of bond in the workplace. Perhaps in some ways, Home Instead felt like a sort of alternate home for me, too.

Hats off to our young new bosses who believed in me and who gave me the creative freedom to promote their business, making my lovely job even better. I tried extra hard for their sakes because it was touching to get such a chance without them micromanaging or monitoring me. In such a workplace, it's no wonder that my passion for working with the elderly stayed alive: I was working with like-minded people who accommodated my needs as I accommodated our clients' requirements.

For Forgiveness and Reconciliation

Having given Bobby credit, perhaps I should also mention the other man who once brought me joy in marriage: Steven. Yes, we had our differences and struggles that ended up splitting us apart, but with Steven, I learned the skills I needed to be a better wife. Moreover, despite our differences, I have to give it to Steven for making our separation and divorce smooth, letting the girls stay with me while supporting them financially. We remained united in our desire to keep them safe and happy.

It took Mr. E to show me what love could look like, Bobby to demonstrate it in reality, and Steven to help me recover from my childhood trauma of my father's abandonment. He proved that not all men are alike in shirking their responsibilities. Perhaps he tried just as hard as I did to make the marriage work, but it didn't because we were destined for other spouses. In any case, for putting our kids first and for making peace a priority, I am grateful to Steven, too.

The Dream That Came True

Finally, I'm grateful for an extremely fulfilling career that satisfied the dream I've had ever since I made that wish back when I was an innocent six-year-old. It taught me to make my life about others and not about myself to find true contentment. In this field, I experienced new things all the time: I explored new cultures and countries and times through my clients' eyes, and I studied and got certifications as I learned about new methods and theories. I explored different families and their pros and cons and learned things I could emulate at home to rebuild my life the way I wanted to see it. I was giving love and receiving it in a balance that helped me feel fulfilled.

My career fulfilled my need to give and care for others, feeling wanted and loved as I gave to those who were alone and helpless. Their happiness was like a balm that warmed my soul.

In a Nutshell: Joys and Gratitude

As I wake up every day, I begin my morning by giving all my praise and thanks to the good Lord for all the ways I've been blessed. I thank him for the ways He made me stand out in the crowd with my unique challenges, toughening me up to become the person I am today.

With the way my life has been, I've grown to appreciate the small things in life that I'd take for granted otherwise and to see my hurdles as advantages that helped me grow. These building blocks paved my path to success and continue to do so today.

In Hindsight

Have you read or heard the bedtime story about the Apple of Contentment? It's about the power of inner peace that can help you through hunger, thirst, grief, injury, and loss. Once you have a taste of it, you can walk through practically anything with a smile because you see beauty and peace everywhere. Such is the power of knowing that everything that happened to you was for a reason and that you are exactly where you need to be.

Looking back at my past and seeing how every event in life helped me learn, grow, or rejoice, my gratitude has no bounds. With gratitude, I believe I can show greater empathy for those who never got the chance to reflect upon their lives and see the beauty in their trials. With those who still have their memories, I can help them see the light of Fate in the hardships that plague them, helping to finally put them at rest.

If I feel gratitude for my life with all its turbulence, I can help others find it, too. Because with it comes a potent peace that puts a smile on your face that runs deeper than the laughter incited by humor. It's a smile of warmth, recognizing at long last that your life was worth living and that you learned and improved.

This is the essence of life that I would like to impart to my clients. Once they have a taste of contentment, it can power them through fits of melancholy, boredom, physical pain, and so much more.

Chapter 10: Tools & Techniques to Treat Dementia

Those with dementia are still people, and they still have stories, and they still have character, and they're all individuals, and they're all unique. And they just need to be interacted with on a human level —Carey Mulligan

There's a difference, I believe, between "just keep them comfortable until the end" and "be a friend to bring them joy while they're still with us." In my years of practice, I've seen both approaches to dealing with the elderly: the first, grudgingly dispensing one's duty, and the second, cherishing the last moments together with love.

I strongly believe in giving the elderly the companionship they deserve when they lose the ability to think wittily, to remember what they last said, and to experience new things. They need someone with the patience to hear the same stories a billion times or to hold their hand and help them remember the way to the park they used to visit every day all of their lives. Not only is it an act of compassion, but it is also something we owe them as a community for having raised our generation.

In short, just because someone has dementia doesn't mean they've lost the ability to laugh or the right to be loved. And these two simple things—laughter and love—lie at the heart of any technique to handle dementia. Let's look at some things I've learned in my years of caregiving. In this chapter, I'll be referring to clients I've discussed in Chapters 2, 3, and 5, in case you've jumped ahead.

The Origins of Care

First things first: You need to have a motive to care for the elderly. Yes, money is a motive. The quality of your care gets you ratings, recommendations, and rankings, and it keeps your house running. However, it cannot inspire you to truly do the best for your client.

Ask yourself: Do your care duties come from a place of love? What brings you to work (or to your elderly relative) every time?

In my case, empathy for the elderly started developing soon after I was born without a left hand. You see, growing up feeling dependent, as if you're a burden or are just existing rather than living, feels terrible. I had a little taste of this, and it was enough that I don't want my clients to ever feel the same way.

Moreover, being abandoned by my father meant that I couldn't bear to watch an elderly person get abandoned. Loving and losing my elderly grandmother and growing up around her friends meant that I grew up cherishing senior people and caring for them.

In short, is there an event in your life that you can use to empathize with your client? Is there a loved one whose memory you can piggyback on to simulate deeper emotions toward your client? Use empathy as your primary tool to work with dementia clients.

With Understanding Comes Compassion

The more you understand about your client, the better you can understand their verbal and non-verbal cues and find the right care routine for them.

In my experience, this begins by having conversations with and observing the client. With Ms. Eileen, for example, it was through observation that I realized she'd lost her verbal filters. After that, I was better prepared with a care routine focused on diversion and damage control.

On another note, I spent a lot of time understanding Mr. E's likes and dislikes. This way, I could use his love for owls to test his memory and his love for children to bring him joy again. In his case, I had to be creative to test his memory and to make him feel needed. Moreover, I had to understand that his "no" didn't mean no; I had to find indirect approaches to what I wanted him to do.

With Mrs. Helen, I needed a great deal of understanding to piece together her life and to make a care routine focused on celebrations because she missed lively events with her loved ones. I had to go along with her thinking that her loved ones were still alive and at home. In her case, memory was the issue, and I needed to deal with it.

With Marie, I couldn't do much because I didn't understand the patterns in her behavior. Although I validated her feelings and offered her time, care, and comfort to ease her suffering, there was little I could do to personalize her care for more effectiveness. Since dementia can affect different people differently, observation and conversation become your next most important tools. Without them, your care routine won't be centered around your clients, and it won't help them as it should.

In short, it's important to unravel the blueprints of who the individual was before this horrible condition took over. Knowing this, I try to understand the client before I develop my person-centered care routine for every unique individual.

Enter Their Stories with Them

As with understanding, it is also necessary to show that you care. This means behaving as more of a companion than a doctor because your job is not to prescribe medicine. *You* are supposed to be the medicine, or you're supposed to incite the laughter and remembrance that can be the medicine.

In Mr. E's case, for example, helping him recall his past systematically and going over his Suitcase of Memories every visit helped him feel better about slowly losing his memories. It helped him feel good about his life. The companionship and sense of fulfillment from my genuinely listening to and enjoying his stories further helped him feel validated and important—like his voice mattered.

With Mrs. Helen, I couldn't really go over her Suitcase of Memories with her because she had lost track of her memories and their order. Instead, I tried to enter the feelings she remembered from those stories, of love and music and dancing and laughter. And as we were loud and happy together, she was able to re-enter those memories in a way that simply repeating them might have utterly failed to do.

In short, as you pay attention to your clients' stories, you get valuable insight into a client's personality while helping them feel heard and cared for.

Laughter as a Medicine

With some clients, you'll find yourself laughing uncontrollably because they're naturally humorous or jolly or because they remember their happier memories. However, you'll often have clients remembering sad or traumatic events from their long lives, falling into melancholy and despondency as they remember these incidents in their loneliness.

With melancholic clients, I try to lighten the mood by adding humorous twists to the memory or situation. For example, with Mr. E I knew I could poke fun at how he jumped from a geologist with "rocks in his head" to becoming a Master Sergeant and then a "carpet man." Similarly, I tried to find humor with other clients so that when they revisit the sadder parts of their lives, they can smile over the funny twists, as well. It's great to uplift their overall mood and quality of life.

Find joy in seeing their smiles; it makes your work fun and their lives a bit happier.

Recreation is Key: Get 'em Outta the House

Yes, I know having the time and money to do whatever you want sounds like a dream, but is it amazing if you're alone and unwell? What do you do when no one needs you outside the house anymore?

With a lot of clients, getting them to places and managing their outdoor activities tends to be a part of the job. This is because, as I found with Mr. E and the slower progress of his mental deterioration, laughter, recreation, and mental stimulation can help immensely.

In Mrs. Helen's case, I was regularly taking her for walks because she loved them. With Mr. E, his love was of food and owls, so I arranged our outings around them. I also planned outings to shopping centers to give him a sense of purpose because he often needed a reason to leave the house again, and sometimes we visited places with old memories like spots for old dates. With Ms. Eileen, our trips were often to her friends' places because she was a social butterfly with an active circle. As you can see, my care routine was planned according to each client's temperament.

In short, I believe in designing outings based on your understanding of your client so that time spent outdoors keeps them engaged and happy rather than stressed and confused.

A Sense of Purpose

When they get old and lose their independence and responsibilities, senior people can feel listless. How do you convince yourself to get out of bed in the morning if you have nothing to live for?

As with Mr. E and pushing Lizzy around in a stroller, giving your clients a sense of purpose in life can truly empower them. Working with Mr. E, the first time I managed to get him out of the house was when I asked him for help getting my daughter a present. The minute I gave him a purpose, his entire attitude changed, and he was ready to embrace life again.

Role Reversals

As you saw in *Teatime with Nana,* Alzheimer's can rob a person of the roles they have had all their lives. For example, when Nana loses the ability to host tea parties, her granddaughter has to host them for her. This is a natural course of action and what an empathetic granddaughter would naturally do.

However, deep down inside somewhere, Nana might still have a sense of loss now that the teatime hosting duties have been taken away from her. It's probably there at the core of her nature, even if she has forgotten how to host. To help people like her, it can sometimes be good to guide them back to who they were before those role reversals. For Nana in the story, for example, it can be helpful if she is guided on how to host parties sometimes. This can give her the feeling that she is caring for her granddaughter, a feeling that has been a part of her nature for a long time, even if she's now forgotten how to do it. This can give her a sense of purpose and bring some of her old traits, if not her memories, back.

In short, do what you can to make your clients feel alive and useful instead of hopeless, empty, bored, or confused.

Old Memories

You might have met someone who can clearly recall events from their childhood and the exact details of their wedding and the hospital where they had their first-born child, but they can't recall what they had for breakfast five minutes ago. In advanced cases, it might look like the client is living in the past or mixing it up with the present.

With such clients, it often helps to bring up some old memories to help anchor them into whatever activity you want them to do. For example, with Mrs. Helen, the problem was with confusing her tenses. However, when I put on the Christmas tree and we danced, I was able to join her in her old memories of happiness and togetherness, making her day. With Mr. E, I often took him to places important to his past. Once, when we visited Coney Island, he came right back to life because it was anchored to memories of his date with Myra.

Whether that memory is tied to an activity, place, story, soundtrack, object, picture, or anything else, use it as much as you can. When your client can't join you in the present, try joining them in their past as you slowly try to bring them out, or even enjoy yourself in their alternate reality!

The Power of Conviction

Have you grown up with strong beliefs or superstitions? Some people, for example, believe that if a black cat crosses the road ahead of them, they'll have bad luck, so they'd rather return home than risk going ahead. Whether it's a religious belief or a superstition, if you practice something for a long period, it can become a part of your subconscious behavior. For an elderly client with Alzheimer's, this can act as something deeply-rooted enough to work with if your client doesn't respond to anything else.

Along with old memories, you can also use your clients' beliefs or superstitions to help them. For example, a devout Christian client is more likely to accept care if you can convince them that it has a religious, biblical element to it. On another note, there is a common superstition for tossing spilled salt over one's shoulder for good luck. If your client has been doing this all their lives, they will remember that it is important to throw that salt over their shoulder even if they can't remember why. Make it a part of your daily exercise routine for them by dropping salt and making them bend, rise, and throw it behind them. Bingo! They'll do the exercise without complaint.

Non-Verbal Cues

Dementia can steal a person's reactions, filters, memories, and behavior patterns. However, once you learn to predict their behavior, you can learn to deal with it.

In this regard, a question I ask myself is, "What do I see when I look into this person's face?"

Of course, there are usual emotions like loneliness, boredom, and despondency. But looking deeper, I can pick out tics. Not everyone is going to shout in pain or say that they're missing their mother; with many, you'll have to watch for extra sadness, extra attachment to a certain object, or something similar for your hint.

There is generally a cue I can identify before, say, a tantrum happens, or when they're hungry but don't remember that they have to eat. Things like wringing their hands, covering their faces, pacing, and any other hints become parts of their behavior patterns that I like to observe so that I can predict their needs and cater to them.

With dementia clients, a lot of what they can't remember to say is there in the non-verbal cues. Pick up on them, and the quality of your care improves drastically.

Non-Verbal Instructions

"Children learn what they live with," they say. They do what others in their surroundings do. Well, senior people are similar to children, just living in the past! And like parents, you'll often have to demonstrate what you want them to do.

As with understanding non-verbal cues, sometimes care can be provided non-verbally, too! You see, the elderly have lived a life where they knew what to do and did things right. Now that they are old and confused, it can be difficult to accept orders or instructions. For example, when I directly asked Mr. E to go outside with me, he refused. Similarly, had I asked Ms. Eileen to stop blaming her friend for her supposedly missing underwear, she might have thrown a tantrum.

In both cases, I needed non-verbal, indirect solutions: In the first case, I pretended that I needed to buy a gift, and in the second, I led by example and made chicken soup as Ms. Eileen and her friend followed, forgetting their argument.

Sometimes, you can get your clients to do things by doing them yourself.

In a Nutshell: Caring in the Time of Dementia

When I see someone with Alzheimer's, I see an individual waiting for someone to connect with. Someone who will understand them and help them reconnect with their purpose and who they once were. They're people who need to have their voices heard and understood, even if they can't articulate those voices or if they get confused halfway.

In Hindsight

As I interacted with more and more clients, I practiced finding the right care plan for each one. With time, I could find patterns across different types of clients. For example, if I'd seen that Mr. E's memory worked better for things he loved, I could test the next client with objects they cherished.

With increased experience and study, I was able to take my caregiving abilities to new levels and found these fundamental tools and techniques to apply to each client.

Chapter 11:
Client Success Stories

The intellect is an inborn quality that increases through knowledge and experience. –Ali ibn Abi Talib

My career as an Alzheimer's caregiver was one where I experienced different cases of Alzheimer's in clients of different backgrounds, memory loss levels, other medical conditions, and life histories. Through it all, I acquired experience. Since 2011, I have been working with even more clients as I stopped being their sole companion. Instead, I oversaw and guided other caregivers who were training under me. This way, I would visit the clients to observe them and to help improve their care plans while I learned from their cases. Add to that the knowledge I gained from my research and accreditation, and my techniques were improving as I went along.

Then, when I started training other caregivers at Home Instead, I realized the importance of demonstrating these techniques through examples I encountered in my career. So, at the end of this book, I'd like to compile some examples from past clients where I'll be breaking down the steps that worked for them.

#1 The Power of Old Memories

After Mr. E passed away, I was given several other clients. I would also have to assist existing caregivers and family members with tools and techniques as I transitioned into my role as a trainer at Home Instead.

A few years after Mr. E passed away, I worked with Mary, a bedridden, 87-year-old Alzheimer's client who was in her final days. She was a former nursery school teacher and a devoted Catholic woman. The caregiver in charge had asked me to observe her and give some pointers to keep Mary engaged and distracted from her pain.

When I arrived, my first step was to try and understand the client, showing her that I was there to help. I held her hand to comfort her and started singing the nursery rhymes I knew, trying to connect with her past self that was still in there somewhere. I wanted to see if those early memories were still accessible and what parts of those memories I could work with. When I got to "Itsy Bitsy Spider," to my surprise, her hands came together to make a spider gesture, moving her hands as if they were spiders. It was an extremely heartwarming moment to see her frail, dejected self come to life as she responded to something after so long.

Encouraged, I looked around Ms. Mary's room for more cues to her past identity. I saw familiar pictures of Catholic saints, Jesus, and Mother Mary, and knew I was in familiar territory, as I had grown up in a firmly Catholic household. I pulled out some rosary beads I found on a countertop, put on the daily mass on TV, and we began reciting and praying with them. As we got into the prayers, I heard a voice: frail, unused, and mumbling, but clear enough to make out the words: "Hail Mary." The lady who had been practically unresponsive for days was not only moving her hands but was also speaking. I was amazed and touched.

Looking at Ms. Mary's example, I realized that the earlier the memory, the better it is stored in the client's mind. With further experience, I solidified what I now call my "Number Line" approach. So, if my client was 87 years old, I could put her life on a number line from 1 to 100. Based on this, I could place her memories from childhood to adulthood.

Now, the client would probably remember nursery rhymes from her childhood, reinforced in her early adulthood when she would keep reciting and repeating them for her students. Therefore, she would remember how to move her hands to the sound, as it was fairly early on the number line.

However, her memory of how to talk could be much further back on the line, so I knew I had to look beyond. Therefore, when I saw signs of devout Catholicism in her room, I knew I could use it as a prop to take her to memories of early childhood because she would have started practicing early on. It would also be a strong memory because she would have continued to practice all the way until she lost track of her memories. Now, when I brought them back in front of her, she could remember the words from those early, deeply stored memories because she was transported to a memory where she prayed aloud. Yes, she couldn't carry on a full conversation because things were blurry, but it was progress, and that was heartening to witness.

In short, when trying to help a client find their memories, I try to find how old they are on that number line. Perhaps Ms. Mary was only four years old on the number line based on her memory, so I had to dig for a memory from that time. See how it works?

Now, as a certified Alzheimer's trainer, I tell my caregivers and aides to bring their imaginary bags to work every day, keeping their clients' Suitcases of Memories in them. These could be from what their clients tell them if their memories are in better shape like Mr. E, or they could be from family members or other sources (like observing the room!) that give hints and insights about the client's past. Every day, they should pull out a story from that bag and use it to transport the client to the right age on the timeline, checking to see which memories they had lost. This way, the client would stay engaged and the caregiver, going back on the number line, could keep track of their memory's progress. Win-win!

#2 Discovering Mystery Triggers

On another visit, I was asked to help with Mr. Smith, an Alzheimer's client who was afraid of showering. He would scream and fight, terrified of getting into the shower. His caregiver was at her wit's end because this was new. He hadn't been afraid of showers before!

Well, in Mr. Smith's case, understanding my client meant going back to that imaginary bag with his Suitcase of Memories. I knew that he was born in Brooklyn, so I could get some cues into his childhood from that. This way, I could tell what he remembered about getting cleaned up when Alzheimer's erased his newer memories and the act of taking comfortable baths became showers to him. And there it was, clear as day: According to his number line, Mr. Smith was still in his early childhood in the 1920s, living in what we call a "cold water flat." Back then, these flats didn't have a heating system for water, so families would boil water until it was a nice temperature. Then, they would bathe in the kitchen or fill a large tub or basin to enjoy a hot bath. While showers had been erased from Mr. Smith's memory, he still remembered hot baths from that time as positive memories. Of course the poor thing was terrified of showers, as they were something he couldn't remember seeing!

Since memories of showers were not in his memory bank anymore, Mr. Smith couldn't be convinced that a shower wouldn't, in fact, be so horrible. He was living in the past. With Mr. Smith, we needed to look for another option: sponge bathing. A bath would bring him back to his earliest memories on the number line where he remembered washing up comfortably. Bingo! He stopped screaming, and the care plan started working for him much better.

You see, sometimes you need to understand the client based on the circumstances they are living in inside their heads. They often don't see the world the same way as you, and logic can't beat their reality. Even if we got Mr. Smith into a warm shower kicking and screaming and logically proved that it was alright, he would forget all about it and go right back to those 1920s memories the next time. As a caregiver or aide, you need to empathize with the fact that old memories have a much longer shelf life than new ones.

At this point, it also becomes important to have a working understanding of other caregiving roles. Officially, I was supposed to provide emotional care, whereas another aide would give the physical care. However, I had learned other bathing techniques (ones that I now impart in the seminars I host), so I could figure out the right way to get Mr. Smith cleaned up without triggering those bad memories.

As I tell my trainees, it's necessary to become a detective and to piece together the client's Suitcases of Memories to figure out their triggers and soothing techniques. You have to unfold their mysteries, place them on their number line, and look for alternative strategies to help find a solution. As a rule of thumb, I teach my trainees that what once worked may not work again on a client with dementia. With the progress of their disease, as they lose more of their memories, the client and their needs keep evolving.

#3 Role Reversals

As a trainer at Home Instead, I was once called to help with Cynthia's client, Dr. Philip, a retired cardiologist. If you recall, Cynthia and I go way back when she was Mr. E's live-in aide, and I was his companion. She had also taken my standard training class for Alzheimer's clients at Home Instead for the companionship aspect of dealing with the elderly. The way she dealt with this case stands out beautifully!

Cynthia was working with a renowned cardiologist, now diagnosed with Alzheimer's. She was keeping him in his Suitcase of Memories, doing her best as an aide and trying to keep his memory active. She had even called me for pointers as his Alzheimer's was getting worse, so you can imagine his state! Dr. Philip was approaching the moderate stage of the disease.

One evening, Cynthia was crying in pain, as her abdomen hurt, and her client saw her. Knowing about role reversals, she took it as an opportunity to help Dr. Philip reconnect with his former duties. She had been trained on the "help me" technique we use in such circumstances. Soon, Cynthia's client was treating her as his patient, bringing out his stethoscope and blood pressure cuff. He took her pulse and continued to care for her until the ambulance arrived.

That night, Cynthia had her gallbladder removed, and her client recalled his skills as a doctor. It was indeed a beautiful night.

As with Cynthia's application of her training, you can see that role reversals can sometimes help clients remember things they seem to have forgotten, especially when they feel desperately needed. It gives them control over the situation, making them remember things. Moreover, perhaps because Cynthia tried to keep Dr. Philips mentally active and in touch with his Suitcase of Memories, he was able to remember so well. A lot of that story truly came to life that night!

#4 Non-Verbal Instructions

Once, on a regular visit to another client called Ruth, I arrived to see her walking out of the bathroom wearing bright pink lipstick - on her eyebrows. Now, to further explain my predicament, we were due for a doctor's appointment, and Ruth was obviously in love with her makeup. Of course, I had to gently clean up Ruth's face and fix her makeup for the time being, telling her she looked beautiful all the same because there was true beauty in seeing her happiness... even if I didn't agree with the cause! I just couldn't let her get laughed at along the way when others saw her appearance.

That afternoon, I brought out two table mirrors: one for her and one for myself. I then limited the amount of stuff on the table, trying to reduce her confusion as to what went where. Next, I put on each cosmetic slowly, letting Ruth copy my actions. So when I applied the eyebrow pencil, she saw what to do and how to do it, and fixed hers up with pencil, too. I made sure that I had my makeup bag with the same makeup items as Ruth, keeping a lipstick, an eyebrow pencil, and a blush. This way, I was able to model the steps with her following along step by step, not using any words. It worked!

As you saw in the previous chapter, helping your clients by leading by example works like a charm without telling them that they are wrong or that they need to learn anything. This way, you don't hurt their feelings or have angry episodes or refusals, streamlining the caregiving process. Secondly, as you saw with the joint makeup session, I used what I call my "Less is More" approach. Essentially, you limit the options to reduce the mental power needed to process everything. Remember, Alzheimer's clients often can't multitask. You have to break down the activity and simplify it for them.

#5 Using the Power of Conviction

On another occasion, I had to help with Ms. Mary, the devout Catholic client I mentioned earlier. This time, she was refusing to take her medication. As Home Instead caregivers, it was our duty to make sure she took the meds on time, but she would struggle, and we couldn't risk hurting her.

Back I went to her Suitcase of Memories, trying to find something that would convince her. Luckily, with Ms. Mary, it was simple: Since she was a stalwart believer in all things Catholic, I could use her conviction that anything to do with religion would be good for her. If you recall, Reader, triggering old memories and the deep-rooted beliefs in them can help reach out to Alzheimer's clients. Therefore, I used the "Body of Christ" approach. This is where you give someone a little wafer called a Host. This is symbolic of the bread eaten at the Last Supper by Jesus and his Apostles, symbolizing the Presence of the Lord. By presenting the meds as a symbol of devotion and reverence to the Lord, I got Ms. Mary to take her meds. Of course, I prayed before using this method because I did not want to be disrespectful, but if it was good for her, I would use her beliefs. It worked like a charm!

At dinner time, I would make sure to use red dishes and red plastic cups. For some reason, probably associated with her past, Ms. Mary would eat better from red containers. Similarly, at dinner time, I would use the "Less is More" approach and limit the amount of food on the dish so that she ate better.

You see, sometimes Alzheimer's can have strange symptoms, and, as caregivers, it is our responsibility to break them down, find out what the client needs, and center the care routine around it. If they're from a different culture or religion, you might have to do research and find out about their convictions. Similarly, you'll have to watch out for slight preferences toward color, shape, size, quantity, et cetera, like a detective to find what works for the client. Plus, doing some research on different types of Alzheimer's and common symptoms to look for can help you guess likely issues in specific circumstances.

#6 A Combination: Recreation, Purpose, and Role Reversals

Once, I was working with John, a 65-year-old retired history professor. He lived with his stepdaughter after his wife passed away at 60 due to breast cancer. John had Parkinson's and was struggling with motor functions and was extremely depressed and lost in life.

I worked with John on some weekends, and he would sometimes call Home Instead, looking for me at work during the week. Just as I did with Mr. E, I centered his care routine around his love for specific activities. With him, it was coffee and museums, so every visit, we would go to a cute, old-fashioned coffee shop where he gave me some excellent history lessons. I would ask him questions about our country, and he loved answering them. This way, he had a sense of purpose, as he was "educating" me, he got his recreation time outside the house, interacting with others, and his mind got its exercise from remembering those facts. I also showed my interest by asking questions and helping him feel needed, as he was helping me. On other occasions, we would visit museums to help him reconnect with old memories and to get a different kind of mental stimulation.

Although John didn't have Alzheimer's, I was still stocking up on his Suitcase of Memories, so I knew that he was grieving for his late wife. He no longer had her to care for and live with. To help with this, I reversed our roles, asking him to help me with cutting my meat, zipping my jacket, and tying my sneakers before our outings. This way, he felt like a man, helping a woman and being needed. John was a wonderful person, and I missed him a great deal after he left for a nursing home out of state.

In John's story, I had to use multiple techniques to care for a client. You see, it will be very rare when a client only needs help feeling needed or just needs someone to drive them out for recreation. As a caregiver, one needs to be aware of different kinds of needs and techniques and merge them for a comprehensive, person-centered care plan.

Steps to Take

Based on the examples above, I can summarize three steps you need to create a person-centered care plan. You'll need to move back and forth through them, though!

1. Create a general Suitcase of Memories based on your research about the client's background. This becomes extra difficult if they or their families can't tell you directly and you just have their religious orientation, place of birth, and similar basic details to work with.

2. Pick out specific details to work with, like the following:

   - Does the client have a super-strong belief about something?

   - How old are they on the number line? Which of their memories would they currently be living in?

   - What reasons does the Suitcase of Memories give for their triggers?

3. Finally, sift through the techniques you've learned (these are just a few!) and pick the right one(s), making a combination to use with the client. For example, you could try the following:

- Is the client feeling useless and dejected? Try giving them something productive to do and give them a sense of purpose.

- If the client is used to caring for others and giving, you could opt for a role reversal and get them to do things for you, replacing the person they used to care for.

- If you need to convince the client to do something, can you get them to follow your actions? Will they quietly take non-verbal instructions and take their meds if you take empty pills, for example?

- Is the client actively struggling and refusing to listen? If this is the case, troubleshoot with the following questions:

    o Can they comprehend what you want them to do?

    o Do they feel you have no right to tell them what to do and are offended or just feeling bullied?

    o Do they feel that you're threatening their control and independence? This is a tricky one because you need to help them without making them feel that you're in control.

    o Is the refusal because they've lost a new set of memories and are confused or disoriented?

- Can you reach out to them with an old memory or conviction to convince them?

- If there is a valid memory the client is reliving that triggers a refusal, is there an alternate care plan you can adopt? Remember, their memories are their reality!

In a Nutshell: Cases That Stood Out

The cases I've given as examples here are just a few from my career as a caregiver and then as a trainer for other caregivers. As you can see, the field can be extremely challenging because every client is unique. In these cases, it looks like you get your Eureka moment instantly. Newsflash: This is absolutely not true! There's a whole lot of trial and error with tantrums and pain until you hit the right routine. You have to go through their history, present medical and mental issues, and their personalities and personalize the plan for each individual client, even though you may struggle desperately with aspects of their behavior you haven't yet figured out until you reach the right conclusions. However, once you reach an equilibrium and start a working relationship with your clients, it's extremely rewarding to see them find some joy in their waning lives and know that you are the reason for their smiles.

In Hindsight

As I said in the previous chapter, care has to come from a place of empathy and love. And despite all the variables and struggles in this profession, I believe that the gratification you get from a job well done where you bring much-needed peace and happiness to the elderly makes it well worth it.

So, at the end of this series, I'd say that my love for Grandma and Mr. E is especially precious because it fueled my care for so many others, helping my love for my clients flourish as an extension. With such strong fuel, I genuinely needed to find quick solutions to help my clients, and that, I feel, made me more successful in thinking out of the box: I just had to do something that would work and work quickly.

Conclusion

*Two roads diverged in a wood, and I—
I took the one less traveled by,
And that has made all the difference.* –Robert Frost

My Suitcase of Memories, just like any other, was colored and molded by the choices I made and the circumstances I faced. Between them, my skills and abilities were molded and colored, too. As I approach the end of this story, I reflect upon how I learned these skills without knowing that I was learning them, how I got through life by giving support and getting it, and only now do I see the extent of their influence on me.

So, with reflection and gratitude, I complete this book and hope that you have found it a relatable story, finding solace in the fact that other's lives, when narrated realistically, are as turbulent as yours likely is or has been. As you chase your own form of stability, I can now say with experience that your stability is also chasing you. All you need to do is stay on track and keep fighting for long enough until you get where you want to be and have clarity.

If you read this book for guidance on becoming a caregiver for someone with Alzheimer's, then I hope the examples of my clients' success stories gave you a glimpse of the creative, innovative thinking you need to work with the elderly. Once you get into the practice, it's both fun and fulfilling to find the right solution. And if you get stuck at any point, I'm always there to help you out!

If you found this sneak peek informative and interesting, hit me up via email for more tips at dementiacareprofessionals@gmail.com. Alternatively, look up my business: It's called Empowering Professionals in Dementia Care, LLC, and it's designed to help anyone watching a loved one or client suffering from any form of dementia. Here, we can work together to find the right solution and explore out-of-the-box options when you've exhausted your regular supply. Sometimes, just talking out the problem can help turn the wheels in your head and lead you to your Eureka moment.

In any case, Reader, I am glad to have shared this journey with you. I hope that whether you picked this book to care for someone or just to read about a real person's story, you found what you were looking for. And if my story helped you, I'd like to request that you pass on the word or leave a review for others who want help or motivation in their respective journeys in life.

To my readers, family, friends, and all those who were with me in my life or in the retelling of my life, I am honored to have had your company and time and am utterly grateful that you shared it with me.

Until the next time we meet, either in a future book, review, or elsewhere, I'm signing off!

References

Beeman, G. (2001). *Smallville - Metamorphosis*. 20th Century Fox.

Bliss, S. (2024, February 25). *Those with dementia are still people and they still have stories and they still have character and....* Medium. https://medium.com/@selfhelpchampion4/those-with-dementia-are-still-people-and-they-still-have-stories-and-they-still-have-character-and-b4b39954b414

Colossians 3:12. (n.d.). *Bible (New International Version)*. https://www.biblegateway.com/passage/?search=Colossians%20 3%3A12&version=NIV

Frost, R. (2024). *The road not taken*. Poetry Foundation. https://www.poetryfoundation.org/poems/44272/the-road-not-taken

Gulpaygani, A. R. (n.d.). *Lesson 3: Natural Disposition (Fiṭrah) and Knowing God*. Al-Islam. https://www.al-islam.org/discursive-theology-volume-1-ali-rabbani-gulpaygani/lesson-3-natural-disposition-fi%E1%B9%ADrah-and-knowing

Hebrews 13:16. (n.d.). *Bible (New International Version)*. https://www.biblegateway.com/passage/?search=Hebrews%2013%3A16&version=NIV

Ingrassia, L. (2004). *Death leaves a heartache no one can heal, love leaves a memory no one can steal.* Her View from Home. https://herviewfromhome.com/death-leaves-a-heartache-no-one-can-heal-love-leaves-a-memory-no-one-can-steal

Jeremiah 29:11. (n.d.). *Bible (New International Version).* https://www.biblegateway.com/passage/?search=Jeremiah+29%3A11&version=NIV

Kaylamalloy. (2023, July 8). *"It's true that we don't know what we've got until we lose it, but it's also true that we don't know what we've been missing until it arrives."* Life's Best Advice. https://lifesbestadvice.com/2023/07/08/its-true-that-we-dont-know-what-weve-got-until-we-lose-it-but-its-also-true-that-we-dont-know-what-weve-been-missing-until-it-arrives/

K., L. (2024). *Poems about hope for the future: A brighter tomorrow through resilience.* The Poeticfy. https://www.thepoeticfy.com/2245/poems-about-hope-for-the-future.

Lunn, K. (2017, October 2). *Poem suggestion - A life well lived.* True Spirit Ceremonies. https://www.truespiritceremonies.com/poem-suggestion-a-life-well-lived

Munshi, P. (2024, July 17). *Top 10 quotes about memories to reflect on your cherished moments with loved ones.* English Jagran. https://english.jagran.com/lifestyle/top-10-quotes-about-memories-to-reflect-on-your-cherished-moments-with-loved-ones-10174112

Phrysylla. (2024). *Echoes of laughter.* Writco. https://writco.in/Poem/P82005072024155220.

Seybold, M. (2016, December 6). *The apocryphal Twain: "The two most important days of your life…"* Center for Mark Twain Studies. https://marktwainstudies.com/the-apocryphal-twain-the-two-most-important-days-of-your-life

Sheers, O. (2005). "The wake". In *Skirrid Hill*.

Sofield, D. (2018, February 4). *Leaving a life imprint.* LinkedIn. https://www.linkedin.com/pulse/leaving-life-imprint-deb-sofield-keynote-speaker

Varma, R. (2023, April 15). *Sunday reflections – On love and life.* Medium. https://rajeev3varma.medium.com/sunday-reflections-on-love-and-life-96e5082f1a78

Watson, L. A. (2015, May 7). *Memories are the key not to the past, but to the future.* Cambridge University Press. https://cambridgeblog.org/2015/05/memories-are-the-key-not-to-the-past-but-to-the-future

Yoon, N. (2016). *The sun is also a star.* Corgi Books.